Weight Training:

How to Lose Weight, Get Rid of Fat, and Keep It Off for Life

Jacob Fits

Table of Contents

Introduction

Obesity has been a growing concern over the years, it's not just about how bad abdominal fat looks it's also about the serious health hazards of carrying extra fat. Even a few extra pounds can cause several health conditions such as hypertension, diabetes, and heart diseases. But sadly, all around us, we see too many people who are unaware or uncaring about these issues.

I am here to help and I want to tell you something, if you are any bit of overweight don't lose hope. You can easily drop it and get in shape quickly.

I want to share a few moves that can help you get the lean body shape you deserve. You can certainly lose fat lifting weights, but we want to go further than that, and get on the fast lane. We want fast results, and so we have decided to compiled other methods and have taken it beyond weight training to achieve better and faster results. By applying these methods together, they are going to give you the best results in the shortest time possible.

Before we begin I'd like to give you a couple quick tips to follow along as we progress through this weight loss journey together.

- Change your diet – Did you know one of the most important things, if not the MOST important thing you can do to lose weight is to change your diet. This is way easier than you might think. Simply by listing your new "diet foods" on your grocery list you will already be preparing yourself for success.

- Eat a lot of fruits and vegetables – This should be on your "diet foods" grocery list. Consuming fruits and vegetables have incredible benefits to them. Besides the energy and nourishment, they provide to the body, vegetables can taste so good when prepared the right way.

- Take adequate fluids throughout the day – Water, water, water. Drink some water, lots of water! Never allow yourself to feel thirsty. The feeling of thirst is your body telling you, you are dehydrated.

- Walk whenever you can – Though, it might be tempting to use the car or call your Uber ride, choosing to walk will only speed up your results. Walking matters and can be transformed into a social activity.

- Go to bed early in the night – Go to sleep as early as you can, the more rest you give to your body, the better your body is going to treat you. Sleeping 7-9 hours per day will leave you feeling refreshed and ready to tackle the world.

As a final note, I'd like to congratulate you for investing in yourself and in your wellbeing by actively moving forward and opening this book. If you enjoy this book, please feel free to let us know on our Facebook page:

Thanks again for allowing us to assist you reach your fitness goals. I hope you reap and benefit greatly from what is inside!

PS.

For your convenience you can skip from chapters to table of contents to get you back to the beginning much faster, in case you are not using a kindle device.

Chapter 1: The Truth About Weight Training for Weight Loss

The thought of weight training to lose weight might seem strange at first, as weight training is associated with building bulk. However, the fact is that, weight training is actually among the best ways to lose all those extra pounds you are carrying around and the best part about it is it works for both men and women.

When you are working to build muscle mass in your body, your muscles will ask for more calories, which you gain from the foods you consume. They will do this because your muscles will require the extra energy for sustenance. This means that your body will now have less calories left over to be accumulated as fat. Your muscles will in short end up eating away part of your body fat.

Even reducing your calorie intake by just a little would improve your results. That is why in order to see your best results, you need to modify your diet plan to ensure that you are consuming fewer calories while you are lifting weight.

However, it's a delicate balance. If you reduce your calorie intake by too much, your muscles will shrink, and this will have the opposite impact. You won't have enough muscle mass to fight the fat in your body. If you are not eating enough, you are essentially making your body starve, causing your brain to go into survival mode, which in turn tells your body to accumulate fat. Your metabolism will slow down, bringing down fat burning as well.

Weight Lifting and Metabolism

To burn fat, you have to increase the rate of your metabolism. You can do this by lifting weights. In fact, your metabolism stays high for several hours after you have left the gym and so you can keep accruing the benefits. When you lift weight, your body needs more oxygen. Your metabolism speeds up to meet this additional demand for oxygen.

Lifting weight flexes your muscles, and this helps with weight loss too. It has been pointed out that muscles can play a key role in increasing your rate of metabolism. In fact, one pound of extra muscle can burn about 20 calories daily.

Weight Training, and the Brain's Hypothalamus

There is another way in which weight training can help you lose fat.

When you lift weight, your heart rate goes up. The heart pumps more rapidly and makes the Leptin hormone in your blood communicates better with the brain's receptor, the hypothalamus. The brain can then send the correct message to your body on whether you should eat more or less. That is, if you are obese, the hypothalamus will tell your body to eat less because it can draw on the stored fat for its energy needs.

For best results you should lift medium weight. After all, you are not trying to become a bodybuilder here. But it would always be better if you combine lifting weights with some cardio exercises. This will help you burn more fat quickly.

Of course, there are many other reasons why you should be lifting weight. For instance, this will boost your endurance and give you stronger bones. Those who lift weight usually sleep better at night too. Researchers have discovered a correlation between weight gain and insomnia. There are quite a few explanations for this. Probably the most logical explanation is that, when the body is at rest, it restores and repairs itself. However, if you are not getting adequate sleep, the fat-metabolizing mechanism of your body won't be able to work efficiently. The bodily organs can work much better when they are well rested. So lift some weights to improve your sleep.

And of course, if you build strength, you will have more energy to carry out physical activities. That's why athletes and bodybuilders spend so many hours in the gym. The extra muscle power will allow you to cycle, swim or run for longer, and this in turn will let you burn more fat without getting tired.

So you see, there is indeed a connection between weight training and weight loss.

Chapter 2: Weight Training to Lose Belly Fat

There's a distinct difference between weight loss and fat loss. The two are not the same. You could be losing weight or burning calories, but there cannot be any guarantee that the weight you have lost is from your fat content.

Weight training helps you lose fat from specific areas of your body, like your belly for instance, as you can target a particular region of the body.

At the very outset, losing weight might seem a simple task. You have to burn more calories than you consume. In reality however, it is more complicated than this. To make sure that what you are losing is fat, you need some control over your hormones.

You need some understanding of the physiology of fat to understand this better.

There are receptors on every fat cell in your body. They are like small keyholes. You have to turn them on to make your cellular machinery lose fat. Hormones are the keys that can open these receptors. There are the catecholamine hormones that work for belly fat. Your body will see several physiological changes when this hormone is docked with its receptor on a fat cell. That's when you decrease muscle loss and burn fat.

You may burn a lot of calories, but it's absolutely essential to stimulate the release of catecholamine for losing fat efficiently. What you need is thus high-intensity weight training.

Human Growth Hormone (HGH) and Lactic Acid

Catecholamine release and intense weight training go together. But the effect of the action of catecholamine on the b-receptors is just the beginning.

When catecholamine is released, it also releases blood sugar. And when you burn sugar through high-intensity activity, the oxygen supply becomes limited. You get lactic acid as a byproduct. When the level of lactic acid goes up, this triggers the release of the Human Growth Hormone or the HGH, and the testosterone hormone. Now HGH and testosterone are two very powerful fat burning hormones.

Testosterone gives you more b-receptors in belly fat. HGH on the other hand prevents the cortisol from storing fat. Working together, these two hormones will let you burn more fat. In fact, once you get this going, you will keep losing belly fat from future workout sessions too.

Study Reveals Amazing Results

The East Carolina University carried out a study recently. The results of this study were published in the Journal of Applied Physiology.

This study revealed that weight training can keep burning your belly fat for hours after you have stopped exercising. Probes were pushed into the subcutaneous fat of the belly in the subjects. The probes remained there, before the training, during it, and up to 15 minutes after the weight training. All the subjects did a complete body resistance-training that included 3 sets of weight lifting and 10 repetitions.

Researchers discovered that the subjects used more abdominal fat during their weight training, and they kept using this for 40 minutes after their exercise.

But that's not the only one…

Another study shows that you can prevent age related fat gain in the abdomen region by doing weight training only two times in a week. The result of this study was presented to the American Heart Association.

The researchers followed 164 overweight women for 2 years. They were divided into two groups. One group was told to do aerobic activities daily for 30 minutes to an hour, while the other group did structure weight-training two times in a week. The second group showed much better results.

Chapter 3 : Weight Training Exercises to Lose Weight

Here are some wonderful weight training exercises you should try.

Barbell Squat

The Barbell squat targets the muscles of your legs. Keep your feet on the floor firmly. Your feet should be planted shoulder-width apart. Now keep a barbell on the upper part of your back comfortably. Avoid your neck. Hold the bar approximately a foot outside your shoulders. Now step out from your barbell rack. Bring your shoulders back and tighten your core. Now squat down slowly till your quadriceps is in parallel position with the ground. Apply pressure to bring yourself up to the standing position. Repeat this exercise after pausing for a couple of seconds.

It is essential to maintain firm position during each squat. Keep your back straight. It shouldn't arch, because there can be a back injury.

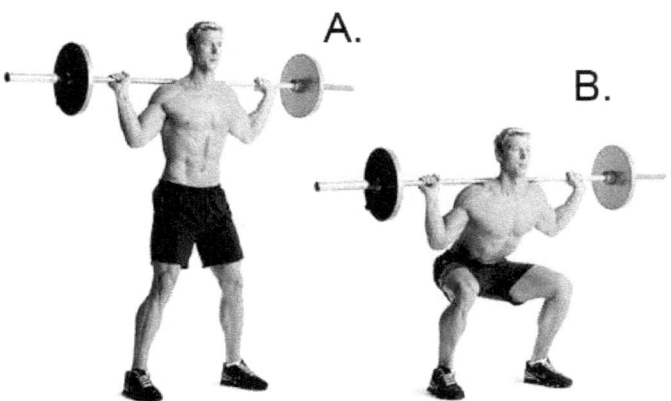

Barbell Squat

Dumbbell Swing

This exercise targets the muscles of your shoulders. Stand a bit wider than shoulder-width. Keep the dumbbell in front of you on the floor. Now squat down. Keep your core tight and hold the dumbbell with your palm. It should face your body. Keep your back absolutely straight as you bring your legs up powerfully. Now swing the dumbbell in the direction of the ceiling till it is at the level of the eye.

Keep your posture strong. Lower this weight down to the floor in a swift and fluid motion. Repeat this 12 times before going to the other arm.

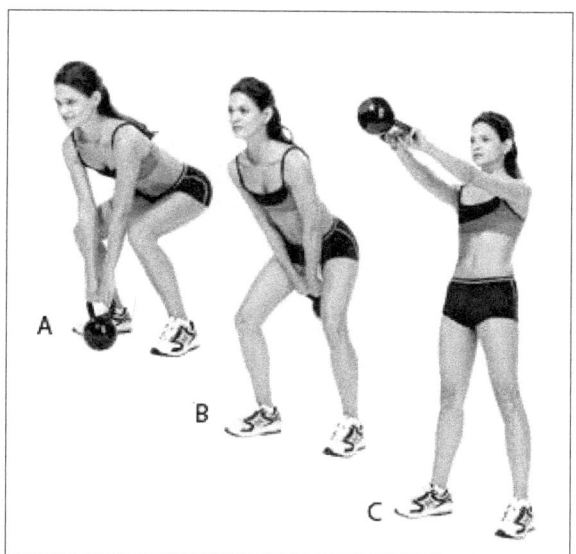

Dumbbell Swing

Dumbbell Front Squat

In the starting position, your feet must be kept shoulder-width apart. Hold a dumbbell in both your hands. Now bring down your body. Make sure that the dumbbells are in front of the shoulders. Your palms should face each other. Your weight should be on your heels. Stop when the hamstrings are in parallel position to the ground. Your core and back should be straight. Keep your chin parallel to the ground. This exercise will strengthen your hamstrings, biceps, and quadriceps. It is easy and very effective.

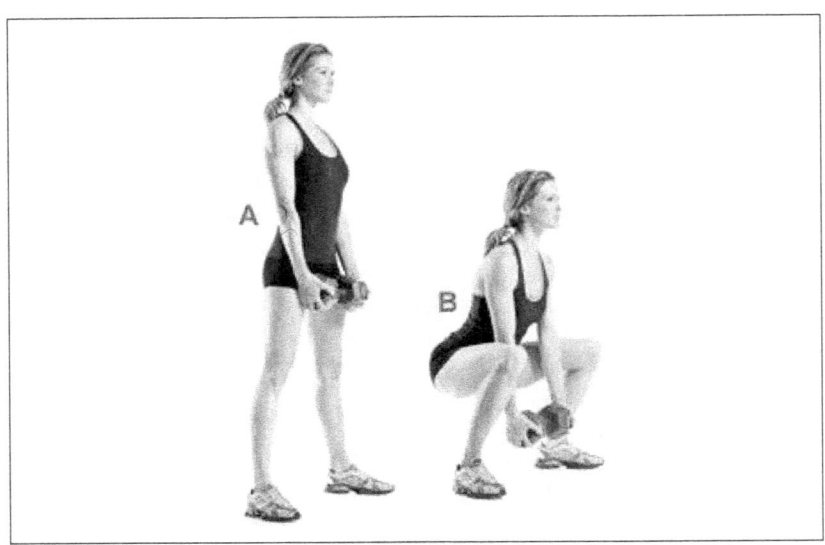

Dumbbell Front Squat

Single-Leg Dumbbell Row

This exercise is for your abs, hamstrings, butt, quadriceps, biceps, shoulders, and back.

Stand straight on the ground, holding a five to ten-pound weight in your left hand. Now hinge forward, making sure that your back is completely flat and parallel to the floor. Get support by holding a low shelf or chair with your right hand. Now extend your left arm towards the floor. Keep your palms facing in Lift your left leg behind you. Your body should form a "T" position.

Bend your left elbow slowly. Bring the weight up till your elbow is in even position with your torso. Lower the weight after holding it for a moment. Do 15 repetitions before switching sides.

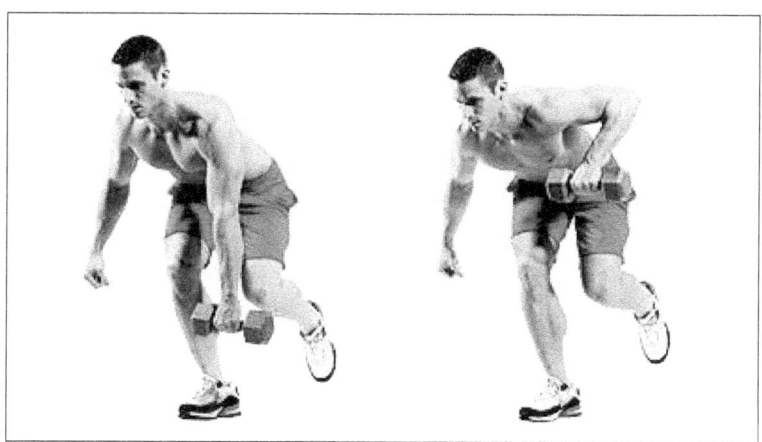

Single-Leg Dumbbell Row

Kettlebell Swings

Kettlebells are balls made of cast iron. There is a single handle in them. Unlike traditional weights that you have to hold, the weight in kettlebells is not distributed evenly. This means that, you have to put in extra effort to stabilize your body so that the balls weight can be counterbalanced.

Use both your hands to hold a kettlebell as your feet is shoulder-width apart. Now extend your arms fully, and squat. The weight should be between your legs. Bring the kettlebell behind and beneath you. Thrust the hips forward, while you swing the weight up to your chest. Your arms should be absolutely straight as you do this. Now lower the weight. Make it pass beneath you. Do a few repetitions. Remember, you must never arch or round your back.

Kettlebell swings are very good because this exercise combines both anaerobic and aerobic activity for burning calories. You will definitely be able to lose weight.

This exercise can be done with a dumbbell too.

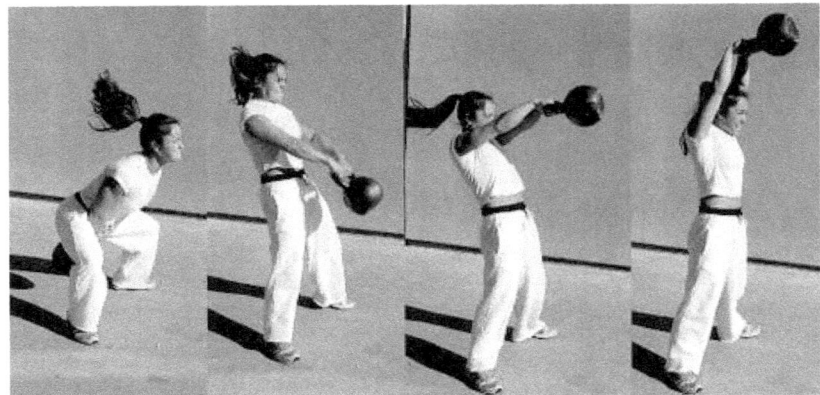

Kettlebell Swings

Squat to Overhead Press

This exercise is for your abs, shoulders, butt, hamstrings, and quadriceps.

Keep your feet shoulder-width apart when you stand. Your elbows should be bent. Hold 5-pound weight in both hands. Keep this weight in the height of your shoulder. Your palms should face forward. Now lower yourself to a squatting position. But make sure that your knees are not going past the toes. Hold this pose and count to three.

Push through your heels for standing up, while you press the weights overhead. Return to the starting position. Repeat 15 times.

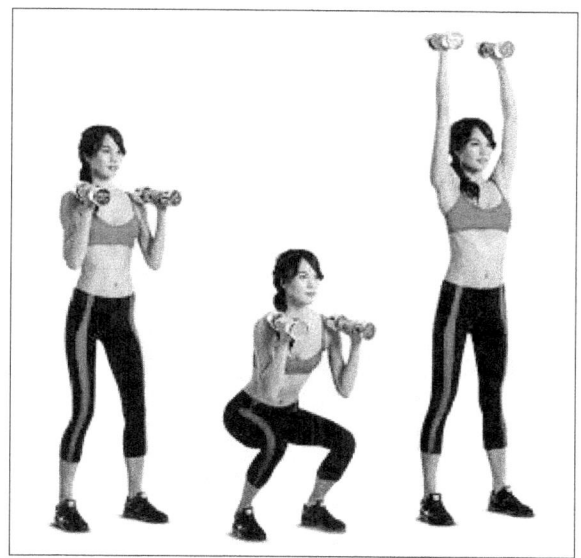

Squat to Overhead Press

Dolphin Plank

This exercise works your abs, shoulders and back muscles.

Lie down on the floor with your face down. Keep your toes tucked. Pull the bellybutton in to your spine even as your forearm is on the floor. Now raise your hips so that they come to the low plank position.

Breathe in while you are lifting your hips. Your body should form the inverted "V" position. Pause for a moment. Return to the starting position. Do three sets of 15 each.

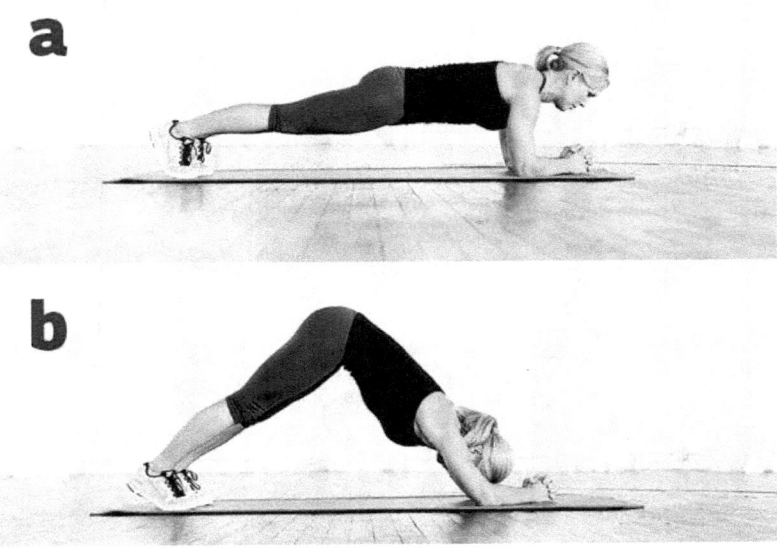

Dolphin Plank

Lower Abs Trifecta

This exercise is for the muscles of your lower abs. It's a great one for losing belly fat and keeping it off for the long-term. It is actually a combination of three lower abs exercises – Reverse Crunches, Ab V Holds, and Ab Pulse Ups.

First do the Abs Pulse Ups. Lie down on your back on a weight-lifting bench or open floor. Keep your hands below your hips if you are doing it on the floor. However, if you are doing this on a bench, then your hands should be below your head. Raise your legs as you tighten your core. Your legs should be in 90-degree angle to your body. Now squeeze your butt and lower abs. push your legs up to your hips. Don't bend your legs. Hold for a second and lower gradually to touch your butt. Do another set. 15 repetitions should be enough.

Move to Reverse Crunches next. Stay on your back and keep your legs in tabletop position. Keep the hands behind your head if you are on the bench. Contract the lower abs and don't move your upper back. Now lift the butts from the floor while bringing the knees to your head. Hold for a second when your knees are chest high. Return to the starting position. You can also put a dumbbell between your feet to make it more difficult.

The next is Abs V Hold. Lie down on your back. Raise your legs and upper body simultaneously even while you contract your abs muscles. Your body should form the "V" shape. Angle between your torso and legs need to be 45 degrees. Keep your legs straight. Your posture should be strong throughout this exercise. Use your hands to hold the knees for as long as you can. Come back to the starting position slowly.

Do these three exercises one after the other without resting.

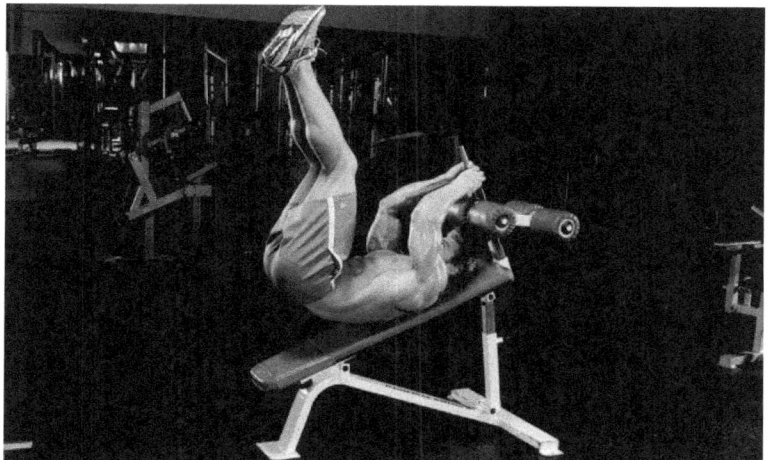

Lower Abs Trifecta

Step-Up with Bicep Curl

Here, you are working the muscles of your biceps, butt, hamstrings, quadriceps, and abs.

Keep your left foot on a bench. Hold 5 pounds' weight in both your hands. Put pressure on your left foot as you try to lift yourself. Keep your right thigh raised so that it is parallel to the floor. Bring the weight up to your shoulders at the same time. Return to the starting position. Switch sides after 15 repetitions. Three sets should be enough.

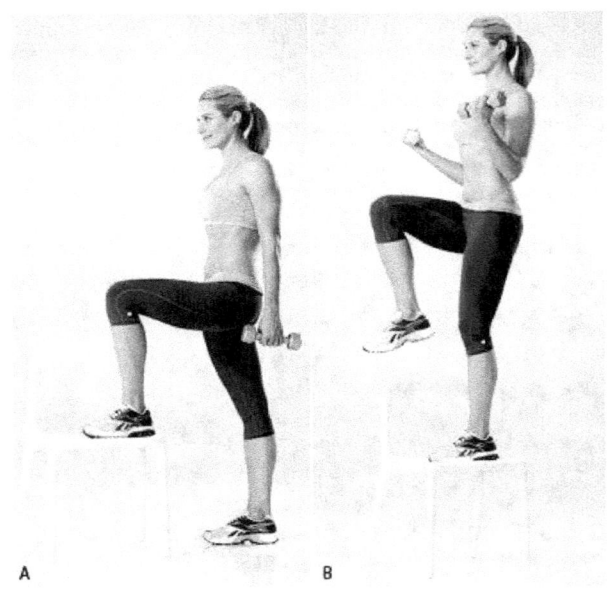

Step-Up with Bicep Curl

Curtsy Lunge

This exercise is for the muscles of your abs, hamstrings, quadriceps, butt, and hips.

Keep your hands on the hip as you stand with feet hip-width apart. Go back a step diagonally with your left foot. Cross this behind the right. Bend your knees when you bring your left hand to the floor. Try to reach the outside part of your right foot with your left hand.

Return to the starting position. Switch sides after doing 15 repetitions. Do three sets of this exercise.

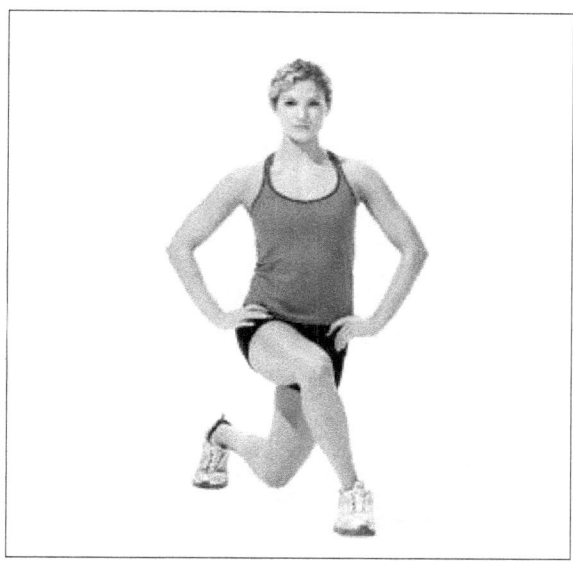

Curtsy Lunge

Cross Fit

Cross Fit is good for people who have been lifting weights for some time. Yes, it can surely help you lose weight, but remember, beginners should still avoid this for later. This exercise involves several workout regimens like endurance exercises, weight lifting, speed and strength training, plyometric, and kettlebell routines among others. You will always stay interested with this one, as Cross Fit is actually several exercises incorporated into one fat-burning workout.

It targets all important physical fitness components, including flexibility, speed, endurance, cardiorespiratory fitness and power.

You can do 30 push-ups, 20 pull-ups, 50 squats, and 40 sit-ups. You can mix it up to make it more interesting. Perform one after the other. Give a 3-minute break between repetitions.

Cross Fit is very effective at burning fat and calories. It improves your endurance, increases metabolism and physical stamina too.

The entire exercise won't take you more than 15 to 20 minutes.

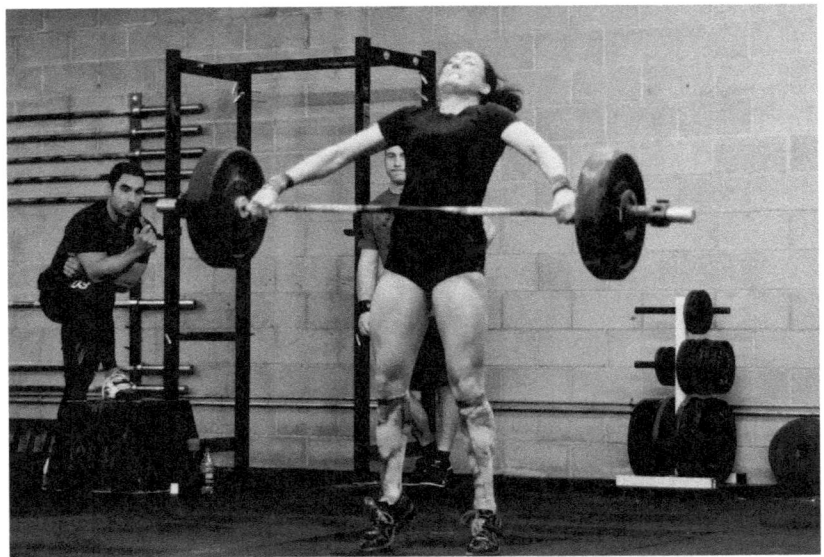

Cross Fit

Turkish Getup

Lie down on your back. Extend your right hand above the chest. Your right foot should stay absolutely flat on the ground. Extend your left leg completely. Keep your left palm on the floor. Now put pressure on the muscles of your abdomen as you sit up. Use your left hand and right foot to get off the ground. Swing your left leg below your body when you lift for maneuvering yourself to the lunge position. Stand up pushing through your heels, while you are moving both your feet side by side. This exercise is good for your core, legs and shoulders.

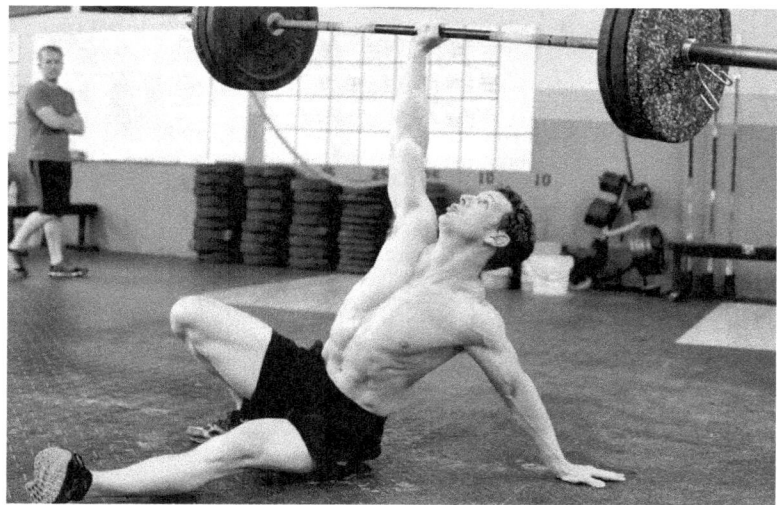

Turkish Getup

Circuit Routine

You can tone the problem areas and burn calories very efficiently by combining free-weight exercises and weight machines. In circuit training, you have to complete each exercise and must take very little rest between them. Here, you are essentially working out on one machine, and then moving on to another without resting for too long, but both are in the same circuit. Finally, spend about 10 minutes on a cardio machine.

Do leg extensions, leg curls, and leg presses for the lower part of your body. Do triceps dumbbell extensions for the backside of your arms, and dumbbell curls for the biceps. Dumbbell military presses should work the muscles of your shoulders. Try side bends and double crunches for the waist. Do 8 to 12 repetitions of each and a total of four rounds. Put on more weight after doing a few repetitions. You will keep losing more fat.

You can do this exercise twice every week.

Chapter 4 : Aerobics for Weight Loss

Weight training can definitely help you get rid of the excess fat. But the fact is that, you can achieve far better results if you add some aerobics and treadmill routines to this. You will not only gain muscle, but the extra effort you are putting in will release all that bottled-up stress as well.

Besides, what are you going to do once you have lost all that belly fat? You need to tone the muscles in your abs. You can do this with aerobics.

In fact, even the Centers for Disease Control and Prevention have recommended aerobics for 3 to 5 hours in a week. You can certainly burn calories and lose weight. But you achieve overall better health as well.

You can do aerobics for 30 to 60 minutes at one stretch or break it up into shorter sessions. But do get your heart pumping and body moving. Vigorous aerobics can help you burn about 500 calories or a pound in an hour.

Step Aerobics

Developed during the late 1980s, step aerobics is low in impact and thus perfect for those who are just starting off. But it will still burn a lot of calories. In a 45-minute session, you can burn as many as 550 calories. That's the same benefits you get by running for 7 miles. With step aerobics, you can target specific muscles on your bum, hips, and legs.

In step aerobics, you will have to use one elevated platform, and thus the name. One foot will always be on the ground or the platform. But do be careful as you can have hurt your knee if your step is too high. Land your entire foot on the step during the exercise. Also make sure that your heel is not extended beyond the edge.

Toning Your Abs

Losing the belly fat is just getting half the work done. You have to make your midsection look attractive. This will increase your self-confidence as well.

Aerobics can tone the muscles of your abs as well and make you look better. Include a couple of strength training exercises in your routine. Each exercise shouldn't take more than 15-20 minutes' maximum. Try ab-toning exercises like the bird-dog. Here, you have to stay on all fours and keep the back flat. Extend your left leg and right arm simultaneously till they are both parallel with the floor. Hold this position. Now stretch your raised leg and arm in opposite directions. Repeat this for 12 times on each side.

Chapter 5 : High-Intensity Interval Training

HIIT or High-Intensity Interval Training is very effective for weight loss. Here, you are essentially alternating between easy and difficult aerobic exercises or simply complete rest, depending on your body condition. In HIIT, the work to rest ratio is between 1:3 and 1:5. For example, if you sprint all out for 30 seconds, then you need to follow it up by walking for 1 minute. Run again for 30 seconds and walk for 2 minutes the second time.

You can do high-intensity interval training on a stationary or elliptical bike, or treadmill. This is going to burn a lot of your calories during the exercise and also after the workout. But remember, HIIT can be quite strenuous for most people. So do this exercise just once in a week and that too for just 20-25 minutes. Don't overdo it because you can get injured.

With HIIT, your body fat might feel like there's no place left for it inside you. It's different than a steady cardio of moderate intensity for 30 to 60 minutes.

Here Are the Results of a Few Studies

1. A study carried out by the Laval University in Quebec, Canada in 1994 found that HIIT was much more effective for fat loss. Young women and men who did High-Intensity Interval Training for 15 weeks lost more fat from their body than those who were on a steady endurance program for 20 weeks.

    This was one of the earliest studies to be carried out. The researchers kept it basic. They divided the subjects into 2 groups and carried out the experiment. One group was made to follow a high intensity interval training schedule, while the other group just did steady-state cardio. Those in the steady-state cardio group actually lost as many as 15,000 calories more than the subjects in the HIIT group. However, subjects in the HIIT group managed to lose more body fat and that too significantly.

2. The East Tennessee State University carried out a study in 2001. This study over 8 weeks showed similar results as well. Subjects were able to reduce their body fat by 2%. Those who did the steady endurance program lost no significant weight.

    This study was titled "A Comparison of the Effects of Interval Training vs. Continuous Training on Weight Loss and Body Composition in Obese Pre-Menopausal Women". The study's purpose was to compare the effects of low intensity steady state training and high intensity interval on body composition and weight loss in obese pre-menopausal women.

All subjects selected, all clinically obese premenopausal women, were divided into two groups. One group was made to do HIIT exercises, while members of the other group did steady state training.

They all had body fat percentage that was greater than or equal to 30%. The subjects were all between the age of 18 and 40. A few of the ladies were between 40 and 45 as well, but they had not yet reached menopause. Subjects were not allowed to make any conscious changes in their eating habits.

The study found that there was no significant difference in weight loss. However, there was indeed fat loss in the group that did high intensity interval training. And so, the researchers agreed that high intensity interval training does indeed cause greater loss of fat mass than low intensity steady training. They concluded by stating that there is a greater reduction in body fat percentage and significant reduction of fat weight. These changes were not observed in the steady state group. The researchers also agreed that high intensity interval training is able to increase muscle mass too.

3. A third study was done in Australia. Female subjects sprinted hard for 8 seconds, and rested for 12 seconds for 20 minutes every day. The group was able to lose six times more body fat.

The University of New South Wales carried out a study on "the effects of high-intensity intermittent exercise training on fat loss and fasting insulin levels of young women" in 2008.

45 female subjects with BMI of 23.2 with the average age of 20.2 years were divided into two groups for the study that was carried out over 15 weeks. At the end, it was discovered that both the groups showed significant improvement in cardiovascular fitness. However, those in the high intensity group showed significant reduction in their total body mass, fat mass, fasting plasma insulin, and trunk fat levels. There was remarkable fat loss in the legs compared to the arms in the HIIT group only. Overweight ladies lost more fat as compared to lead women. The researchers concluded by saying that high intensity interval training done correctly 3 times a week for 15 weeks was able to reduce significantly more body fat, trunk fat, and improve insulin resistance among young women.

4. We also get important insight from another study that was carried out by The University of Western Ontario. From this study, we can learn how effective high intensity interval training really is.

Researchers here, divided the subjects into two groups, and had 10 women and 10 men train thrice in a week. The first group did between 4 and 6, 30 second treadmill sprints and tool between 4 and 6-minute rest between each. The second group did 30 to 60 minutes of steady-state cardio.

After training for 6 weeks, the subjects who were on interval training showed much more weight loss. So it can be said that yes, you can burn more fat with HIIT than doing an inclined treadmill for 60 seconds.

To be completely honest, the exact way in which high intensity is able to beat cardio isn't understood completely yet. However, having said this, researchers have managed to isolate several key factors. They are,

- Higher resting metabolism up to 24 hours after the workout session.

- Higher fat oxidation level in the muscles.

- Better insulin sensitivity in the muscles.

- Increases level of HGH or the Human Growth Hormone, which incidentally can help you lose weight as well, and increased catecholamine levels as well. Catecholamines are chemicals in the body that induces fat mobilization directly.

- Appetite suppression after exercise.

5. The Baylor College of Medicine at Houston carried out their study in 1996. At the end, the researchers reported that subjects on the HIIT regimen were able to burn appreciably more calories in 24 hours after the workout, as compared to those who were on steady state intensity. This happened because of an increase in their resting metabolism. High intensity interval training is tougher on the body. Your body will have to put in more energy to repair itself after the exercise, and this is what will make you lose more calories.

   Incidentally, the study carried out by East Tennessee also discovered that subjects lost 100 calories more for up to 24 hours after the exercise.

6. More recently, the Florida State University at Tallahassee also carried out their research. Its findings were presented at the Annual Meeting of the American College of Sports Medicine in 2007. According to the findings, subjects on high intensity training were able to burn 10% more calories for up to 24 hours after the exercise, as compared to those who were in the steady state group.

6 Ways in Which HIIT Can Help Your Weight Loss Efforts

We all want quick results, and ideally, we don't want to scrutinize every meal we have or spend hours at the health club so that we can lose a pound after a month of hard work. Yes, it is true that there is no magic pill that can give you overnight results, but having said this, you can still lose weight quicker through HIIT or high intensity interval training.

Most average people don't know about HIIT. This method is actually followed by endurance athletes and fitness models to improve their metabolism and melt the fat away quickly before a competition. Many consider this to be the most effective cardio workout that can be performed in 30 minutes or so. And the best part is, you can do most of these exercises almost anywhere.

Another great thing about HIIT is that, you will be able to customize it for your own needs and body type, and can still get the desired results. So you can certainly do HIIT. The only exception is those with arthritis or heart problems.

Here are some common exercises in high intensity interval training...

- Jumping Rope
- Running
- Swimming
- Lunges
- Burpees
- Running up stairs
- Knee-ups
- Push-ups
- Jumping Jacks
- Yoga Balls
- Kettle Bells

The 6 Benefits of HIIT

1. Burns fat quickly and keeps it away – According to the results of a study conducted by the East Tennessee State University (details mentioned above), subjects were able to lose 2% more body fat with high intensity training, as compared to others. In fact, the subjects managed to lose as much as 100 more calories every day.

   It was also found that if you do HIIT, you can even burn calories just by sleeping or sitting after a workout session. This means, you will keep losing weight even when you are not exercising. No wonder, so many fitness fanatics and athletes are into high intensity training.

2. Saves you time – Most of the equipment needed for these exercises are there in most gyms, such as an elliptical or treadmill. And for some of these exercises, you won't require any equipment at all. In so many gyms, you will find people slogging it out for weeks and months, hoping to lose a few pounds. They become physical tired and mentally exhausted, and often quit, as the results are slow. Not with HIIT. Yes, the exercises will drain your body and you will feel tired, but you

will remain mentally charged-up, as the results are quick. It's just for a few weeks, and so you can keep yourself going. HIIT takes just 40 minutes of your time daily, and that too for just 3 to 4 days in a week. No more! You won't have to spend so many hours in the gym again.

3. You can do these exercises almost anywhere – Here is another great benefit. Do you have a track close to your home, or a swimming pool? Perhaps you have a little bit of extra space in the basement or one of the rooms in your house. That will do. You can do the high intensity training exercises at any of these places.

   There could be a snow storm raging outside, preventing you from going to the gym. No issues! All you have to do is just wear comfortable exercise clothes and do these exercises at your home or the track close to your place. Often, you don't even need the elliptical machine or the treadmill. You can use them if you have them. But there are other options too.

   You can keep it interesting as well, as there is a lot of variety in these exercises. You are always switching over from one to another. The fact is that, quite often, many individuals quit as they get bored from their workout regimen. There is very little chance of this happening here.

4. Endurance – You will find a few people who are skeptic about HIIT, but, trainers, competitors and athletes will all vouch for this. They will tell you that, apart from helping you lose weight, high intensity training can also help you improve endurance. Endurance is important in a long race. But it's going to help you otherwise too, even if you are not planning to sign up for a race or cross obstacles. With these exercises, you can overcome dizziness, muscle cramps and shortness of breath. Your body will be in much better shape to fight the fat accumulation. And this is certain to help you in your endeavor.

5. Helps you preserve muscle mass – Doing cardio exercises all the time isn't going to help you lose weight. HIIT is going to reduce the chance that your body is going to use the muscles as fuel. This ensures that you can preserve the mass, something that isn't going to happen with regular sessions of cardio. You can maintain strength if you can conserve your muscles. This will give you better endurance too.

   Studies have revealed that apart from reducing fat, the muscle fibers of subjects who did high intensity interval training had had more markers for fat burning than those who were just on cardio. Cardio can certainly help you burn calories, but with this, you will lose muscle mass too. But that's not going to happen with HIIT.

6. Gives you results quicker than traditional cardio – In high intensity interval training, you will be stopping and going constantly, and pushing your body to the maximum. And so, you will be using much more energy than somebody who is just running 5 miles in an hour. You will eventually be speeding up your metabolism. These exercises will stimulate the production of HGH or Human Growth Hormone by over 450%, and this will stay with you up to 24 hours after

you have completed doing the exercises. As a result, you will keep burning fat, even after completing the workout session. Over time, you are going to burn fat much faster as compared to traditional cardio.

But having said this, you will still need to change your diet. High intensity interval training is always going to be most effective if you are on a healthy diet plan. So make sure that you are having plenty of green vegetables, rich carbohydrates and lean meat. Stay away from all those greasy and fatty fast foods and cola drinks.

High Intensity Interval Training Procedures

Peter Coe Regimen – This is high intensity interval training where there are short recovery periods. This was first recommended during the 1970s by Peter Coe, who was an athletics coach when he was planning exercise sessions for his son Sebastian Coe. Peter was inspired by the principles of Woldemar Gerschler, who was a university professor and coach from Germany, and Per-Olof Astrand, the physiologist from Sweden. Peter planned sessions with fast 200 meter runs that were repeated in cycles. His son could rest for just 30 seconds between two fast run sessions.

Tabata Regimen – This procedure was based on a study conducted by Professor Izumi Tabata in 1996 for Olympic speed skaters. Here, there were ultra-intense exercises for 20 seconds, which was followed by rests for 10 seconds. The participant had to complete a total of 8 cycles in 4 minutes. Exercises were done on a cycle ergometer with a mechanical brake. Tabata named it the IE1 protocol.

Athletes who followed this regimen, trained for four times in a week. The fifth day was spent doing steady-state training. Tabata found that with this method, the athletes were able to gain more overall.

Gibala Regimen - Professor Martin Gibala from the McMaster University in Canada and his team was busy researching high intensity interval training for many years. They carried out a study in 2009 on students in 2009. They were made to warm-up for 3 minutes, and then do intensive training for 60 seconds, which was followed up by rest for 75 seconds. Each student had to repeat this cycle between 8 and 12 times, depending on individual ability. The students trained for 3 times in a week. A less intense version of the regimen was published later by Gibala in 2011. Both these versions provide very good results.

Timmons Regimen – Jamie Timmons was a systems biology professor at the University of Loughborough. He came out with this regimen involving a few short bursts of flat-out intense exercises. In a program on BBC Horizon in 2012, Jamie put Michael Mosley on an exercise bike. Mosley had to do 3 sets of gentle pedaling for 2 minutes each, and then a cycling burst for 20 seconds where he gave maximum effort. The set was for a total of 21 minutes, and was performed thrice a week. This included warm-up and recovery time.

10 Rules for High-Intensity Interval Training

Rule #1 – The interval workout session should give your body a serious jolt between 10 and 40 minutes.

- The workout session should be so intense that you won't feel like doing anything else once it is over. You will feel like just relaxing for half an hour. But of course, you should be able to carry out simple tasks such as walking at normal pace.

- Make sure that the workout is never easy. In other words, it should be seriously challenging. In fact, it needs to be so challenging that doing it for 40 minutes seems impossible to you. It's possible that you might not be able to do it for 40 minutes in the beginning. That's fine. Keep trying, and you will see that your performance will improve slowly.

- Basically, the interval training session needs to scare you. But somehow, you must still summon up all the courage to complete it, as interval training will certainly help you shed those excess pounds quickly.

Rule #2 – The hardest parts of interval training shouldn't take up a lot of the 40 minutes. You can break up the most difficult exercises into smaller segments of 60 seconds each.

Rule #3 – But do keep in mind that the easier parts of the interval training workout session shouldn't be more than double the time of the hardest parts.

- For instance, if you do the "Jumping Jack Interval Workout", where you are doing jumping jacks for 20 seconds, then make sure that you are doing this as fast as you can. That would increase the challenge and would be the difficult part.

- After this, don't rest for more than 40 seconds. This is your easy part. Now get back to doing jumping jacks again as fast as you can. Do this exercise for another 20 seconds. So once more, you return to the hard part.

Rule #4 – The hard parts of the interval workout should be "really" hard.

- For instance, is you have a scale of 1 to 10, then make sure that your interval workout is somewhere at 11. That's how difficult the hardest parts of the exercises need to be.

- In fact, the hardest parts should be so difficult that you will actually be waiting for the easier parts so that you can get the badly needed rest. That would mean that you are doing it good.

- The hardest parts should be so intense that you will not even feel like talking to anybody. You should have to give 100% of your focus so that you can give maximum efforts for these 40 seconds.

Rule #5 – Yes, the hardest parts of the exercises will be very difficult, but you need to make sure that the easier parts are actually really "easy".

- You should be at 1, on a scale of 1 to 10. In other words, in the easier sections, you should be very close to actually doing nothing at all.

Rule #6 – Do remember, you should not, under any circumstances, do high intensity interval training for more than 3 to 4 days in a week.

However, having said this, you can lose as much as 15 lbs every 3 weeks if you break this rule. But you have to keep in mind a few things before breaking this rule.

- Always make sure that your interval workouts are really exerting yourself for the 3 to 4 days in a week when you are doing them.

- If the interval workouts are not really extremely challenging, then you will have to find ways of making the sessions more intense. That's because, you need to seriously challenge your body if you are going to relax for 3-4 days in a week. See rule 10 to discover how you can make the sessions more difficult.

- If your sessions are intense enough, then anyway, for most people, it would be impossible to do interval training for more than 3 to 4 days in a week unless you are desperate to lose weight really fast.

Rule #7 – If you are doing other exercises too, then make sure that your interval sessions are always "last".

- Always do the muscle building or toning exercises for burning fat before your interval training sessions.

- That's because, high intensity interval sessions, if done correctly, are likely to be so difficult that you won't be left with any energy for these other exercises once you have done them.

Rule #8 – If you can manage it, then you must do interval training twice a day for the 3 to 4 days in a week. That is going to give you much better results. You will see that you are losing weight more quickly. However, this is optional. Everything depends on how well your body is able to take it.

- You can try doing the interval training right in the morning before your breakfast. The second session can be done in the evening. By spacing it in this way, you will be giving your body enough time to recover.

- The 20 to 40 minute sessions of interval training are so intense that ideally, your body needs rest for anything between 2 to 4 hours in between two sessions in a day.

- In fact, you may even do interval training more than twice in a day. But for this, make sure that each session is not more than 10 minutes.

Rule #9 – You have to alternate between upper and lower body interval training.

- When you begin to do the interval exercises, make sure that you are alternating between the lower body such as the elliptical workout, and exercises for the upper body such as the sledgehammer workout.

- For instance, if your lower body is tired from the elliptical workout, then you can switch over to the sledgehammer workout for your upper body. In this way, you can still give your 100% and won't have to worry about your upper or lower body unable to take it anymore.

- You should face no problems in alternating between upper body and lower body workouts when you have become fit enough.

Rule #10 – Always make a serious effort to beat your performance in the last session. This is the right approach. This is the way to challenge your body.

- For instance, if you gave 85% effort in the last session, then make a conscious effort to give at least 86%. Every little bit helps.

- It is OK if you cannot exert yourself a bit more. There is always going to be a next time. But having said this, you must also ensure that you are not slacking off too much, and ending up giving 75%, as every time you do interval training, ideally, you have to push yourself slightly more. That's the way to keep burning more fat.

5 Ways of Beating Your Last Interval Training Workout Session

I have said before, that have to make each session intense, and not just that, each session has to be more intense than the last one. Here are 5 ways in which you can do this.

1. Make the easier parts of the workout shorter, or rest for less time after the hardest phase of your interval training.

2. Try to extend the hardest parts of your exercise extend beyond 40 seconds.

3. If you think your body can manage it, then try and continue doing interval training for more than 40 minutes.

4. Make the hard part even harder. You can do this by walking on an incline, walking or running faster, or by wearing a weight vest.

5. Maintain a weight loss workout log. This will help you track how many calories you have burned, how fast you went during the exercise, or how many miles you were able to complete. You will then have data that you can try to beat in your next interval training session.

8 Extremely Effective Fat-Burning Interval Training Exercises

Workout #1

This exercise consists of 4 rounds.

Round One:

- Burpees.
- Mountain Climbers.
- Jumping Jacks.

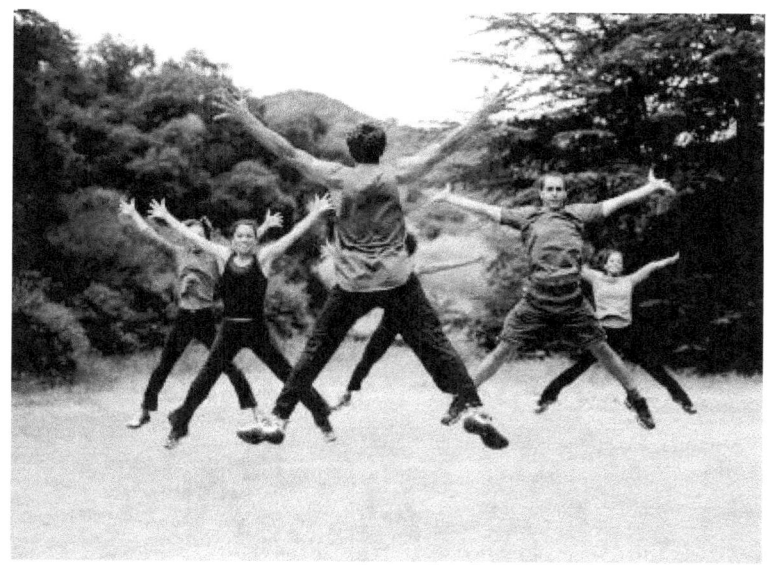

Jumping Jacks

You must do 3 circuits – 10 reps in the first round, 15 reps in the second round, and 20 reps in the third round. You cannot stop in between. No rests.

Jump rope for 3 minutes. Rest for 1 minute.

Round Two:

- Walking Lunges with Kettlebell exchange below the leg.
- Pushups.
- Lunge Jumps.
- Walk-outs.

You have to do 3 circuits – 45 seconds for each exercise. Take a break for 15 seconds between each exercise and circuit.

Jump rope for 3 minutes. Rest for 1 minute.

Round Three:

- Traveling Kettlebell Squats.
- TRX Pull-ups.
- Box Jumps.
- TRX Jack Knives.

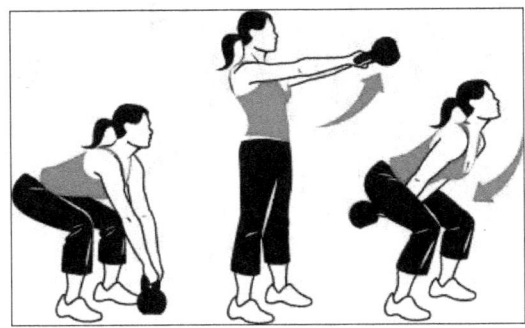

Kettlebell Squats

You must do 3 circuits – 45 seconds for each exercise. Take a break for 15 seconds between each exercise and circuit.

Jump rope for 3 minutes. Rest for 1 minute.

Round Four:

- Traveling Side Lunges.
- Dips.
- Speed Skaters (lateral jumps).
- Plank to Pushup.

You must do 3 circuits – 45 seconds for each exercise. Take a break for 15 seconds between each exercise and circuit.

Workout #2

- Jump Rope.
- Plyo Push-up.
- Bodyweight Rows.
- Medicine Ball Squat to Overhead Throw.
- Burpee.
- Medicine Ball Chest Pass.
- Renegade Rows.
- Jumping Lunges.
- Planks.
- Treadmill Incline Sprints.

Here, you have to exercise for 20 seconds and then rest for 10 seconds for each exercise mentioned above. Do each of them once, one after the other, and then repeat the entire circuit. But remember to rest for a couple of minutes before repeating. Your aim should be to complete three circuits.

Workout #3

This is a strength and conditioning exercise with battling ropes.

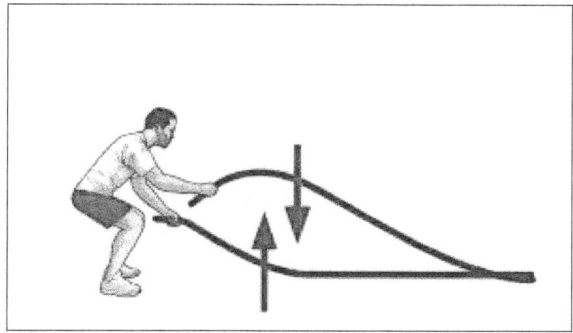

Battling Ropes

Do this exercise for 30 seconds. Try to move the rope 25 times in this time.

Now take rest for 15 seconds.

Do the sledgehammer exercise to a tire for 30 seconds. Hit the tire as fast as you can.

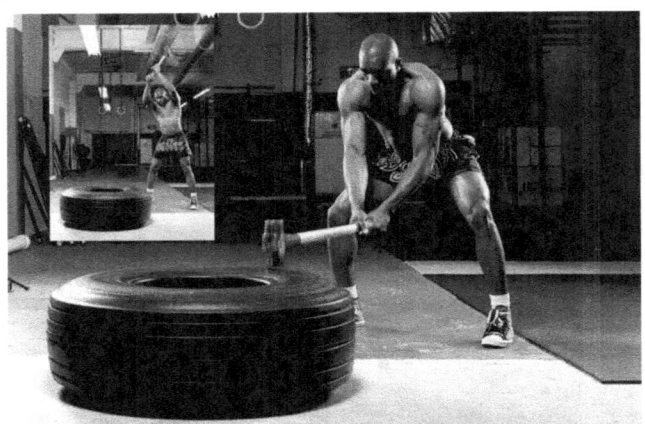

Sledgehammer Exercise

Take rest for 60 seconds after this.

Repeat the set for a couple of times.

Workout #4

Do the loaded sled push exercise. Push it 30 yards.

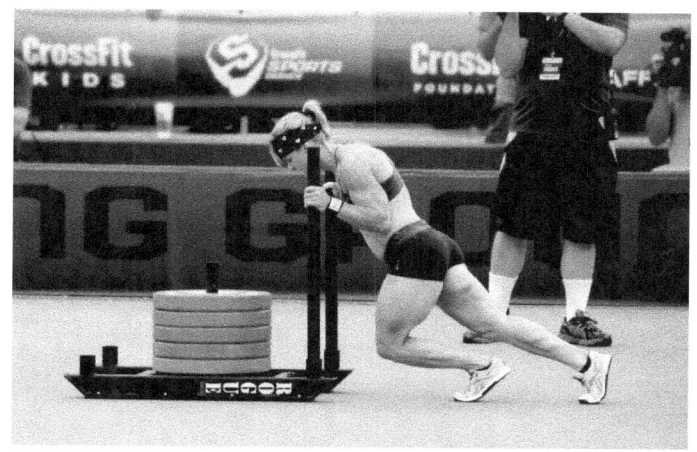

Sled Pushing Exercise

Do 25 Kettlebell Swings after this.

Take rest for 90 seconds between two sets.

Repeat this 2 to 3 times.

Workout #5

This is a simple one. Begin by sprinting for 1 minute. Try to sprint as fast as you can. Rest for 90 seconds once you have completed sprinting for a minute.

Now sprint for 1 minute at 3% incline to make it more difficult for you. Rest for 90 seconds like before.

Sprint for 1 minute at 6% incline, and rest for 90 seconds once completed.

Sprint for 1 minute at 9% incline and rest for 90 seconds.

Make it even more difficult by sprinting at 12% incline. Rest for 90 seconds for recovery.

Repeat the entire set 3 to 6 times, depending on how well your body is able to take it. But try to improve your performance. For instance, if you could do 3 sets on the first couple of days, then make a conscious effort to reach at least 5 sets by the end of the second week.

Workout #6

Jog for 5 minutes. This will be your warm up.

Now increase the speed or intensity till there is a significant increase in your heart rate.

Now lower the intensity to brisk walking or just a jog till the time your heart rate slows down quite a bit. Jog for 5 minutes to cool down.

To begin with, you have to do this interval training for anything between 4 and 6 rounds.

Set a time limit when conditioning increases, and try to achieve a goal. Get a heart rate monitor if you can. If you cannot, then count your pulse for 6 seconds. Now multiply the number by 10. You will be able to find your heart rate.

Workout #7

- Tire Flips for 30 seconds.
- Medicine Ball Slam for 30 seconds.
- Battle Rope Slams for 30 seconds.
- Loaded Sled Push – 100 yards.
- Farmer's Walk – 100 yards.

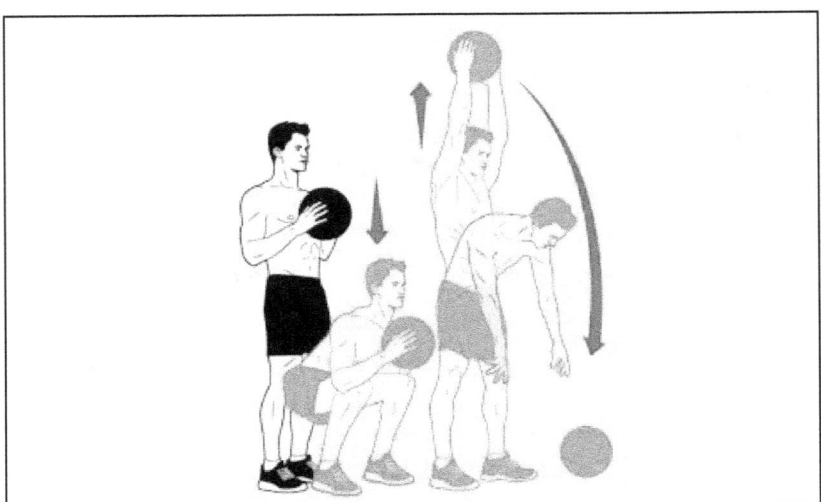

Medicine Ball Slam

Repeat the set for 4 rounds. But make sure to rest for 2 minutes between each round.

Workout #8

- Kettlebell Swings for 30 seconds.
- Right Arm Kettlebell Snatch for 30 seconds.
- Right Arm Kettlebell Push Press for 30 seconds.
- Right Arm Overhead Walking Lunges with Kettlebell for 30 seconds.
- Sprint for 30 seconds.

Rest for 90 seconds after completing this entire set. Now repeat this on your left arm. Your aim should be to complete 2 to 3 sets for each arm.

Beginner, Intermediate, and Advanced Level Interval Training

A. Beginner weight loss interval routines

1. **Basic interval workout**
- Begin this by warming up for 3 to 5 minutes.
- Now do a high intensity activity for 20 to 45 seconds.
- Switch over to a low intensity workout for 60 to 90 seconds. Alternatively, you may decide to do nothing and just rest as well.
- Repeat this schedule for 10 to 30 minutes.

Here is one good example of a basic interval exercise...

- Start by warming up for 3 to 5 minutes.
- Run on a treadmill for 20 to 45 seconds. You should run at no slower than 7 miles per hour.

- Switch over to walking on the treadmill at 2 miles per hour. Walk for 60 to 90 seconds.
- Repeat this for 10 to 30 minutes.

Here is one more example of a basic interval exercise...

- Start by warming up for 3 to 5 minutes.
- Get up on a treadmill and walk fast at 5 miles per hour for 20 to 45 seconds.
- Walk slowly at 3 miles per hour for 60 to 90 seconds.
- Repeat this for 10 to 30 minutes.

2. **Pyramid Interval Workout**

- Start by warming up for 3 to 5 minutes.
- Do a low intensity exercise for 1 minute or rest completely – do nothing.
- Become much more active. High intensity exercise for 30 seconds.
- Once again, complete rest for 1 minute or a low intensity exercise.
- Switch over to a high intensity activity for 30 to 45 seconds.
- Complete rest for 1 minute or a low intensity exercise.
- High intensity activity for 40 to 60 seconds.
- Low intensity exercise or rest for 2 minutes.
- High intensity exercise for 40 to 60 seconds.
- Low intensity exercise or rest for 1 minute.
- High intensity exercise for 30 to 45 seconds.
- Low intensity exercise or rest for 1 minute.
- High intensity exercise for 30 seconds.
- Low intensity exercise or rest for 1 minute.
- High intensity exercise for 30 seconds.
- Low intensity exercise or rest for 1 minute.

- High intensity exercise for 30 to 45 seconds.

- Low intensity exercise or rest for 1 minute.

- High intensity exercise for 40 to 60 seconds.

- Low intensity exercise or rest for 2 minutes.

- High intensity exercise for 40 to 60 seconds.

- Low intensity exercise or rest for 1 minute.

- High intensity exercise for 30 to 45 seconds.

Stop here if your interval workout is for 20 minutes. Or else,

- High intensity exercise for 30 seconds.

- Low intensity exercise or rest for 1 minute.

- High intensity exercise for 30 to 45 seconds.

- Low intensity exercise or rest for 1 minute.

- High intensity exercise for 40 to 60 seconds.

- Low intensity exercise or rest for 2 minutes.

- High intensity exercise for 40 to 60 seconds.

- Low intensity exercise or rest for 1 minute.

- High intensity exercise for 30 to 45 seconds.

- Low intensity exercise or rest for 1 minute.

Stop here if your interval workout is for 30 minutes.

Here is one more example of the Pyramid Interval Exercise…

- Start by warming up for 3 to 5 minutes.

- Ride a stationary bike slowly for 1 minute.

- Ride a stationary bike quickly for 30 seconds.

- Ride a stationary bike slowly for 1 minute.

- Ride a stationary bike quickly for 45 seconds.

- Ride a stationary bike slowly for 1 minute.
- Ride a stationary bike quickly for 60 seconds.
- Ride a stationary bike slowly for 2 minutes.
- Ride a stationary bike quickly for 60 seconds.
- Ride a stationary bike slowly for 1 minute.
- Ride a stationary bike quickly for 45 seconds.
- Ride a stationary bike slowly for 1 minute.
- Ride a stationary bike quickly for 30 seconds.
- Ride a stationary bike slowly for 1 minute.
- Ride a stationary bike quickly for 30 seconds.
- Ride a stationary bike slowly for 1 minute.
- Ride a stationary bike quickly for 45 seconds.
- Ride a stationary bike slowly for 1 minute.
- Ride a stationary bike quickly for 60 seconds.
- Ride a stationary bike slowly for 2 minutes.
- Ride a stationary bike quickly for 60 seconds.
- Ride a stationary bike slowly for 1 minute.
- Ride a stationary bike quickly for 45 seconds.

Stop here if your interval training is for 20 minutes. Or else,

- Ride a stationary bike slowly for 1 minute.
- Ride a stationary bike quickly for 30 seconds.
- Ride a stationary bike slowly for 1 minute.
- Ride a stationary bike quickly for 45 seconds.
- Ride a stationary bike slowly for 1 minute.
- Ride a stationary bike quickly for 60 seconds.

- Ride a stationary bike slowly for 2 minutes.
- Ride a stationary bike quickly for 60 seconds.
- Ride a stationary bike slowly for 1 minute.
- Ride a stationary bike quickly for 45 seconds.
- Ride a stationary bike slowly for 1 minute.

Stop here if your interval training is for 30 minutes.

B. Intermediate weight loss interval routine on hill or stair

For the stair or hill interval training for weight loss,

- You have to walk up and down a hill, which is minimum 50 yards, or,
- You must walk up and down a minimum of 4 flights of stairs for anything between 10 to 30 minutes.
- Walking up the stairs or hill is the high intensity part of the exercise.
- Walking down the stairs or hill is the low intensity part of the exercise.

For those who are close to the beginner level...

- Jog or walk up a hill. Rest for 30 seconds once you have reached the top. Begin to walk down after this. Keep repeating this schedule for 20 to 45 minutes, or,
- Jog or walk minimum 4 flights of stairs. Walk down the stairs or you can take the elevator as well. Keep repeating this for 20 to 45 minutes.

For those who are truly in the intermediate level...

- Run or walk up and down the hill for 20 to 30 minutes, or,
- Run or walk up and down the flight of stairs for 20 to 30 minutes.

For those who are close to the advanced level...

- Sprint, run or jog up the hill. Now walk back. Keep doing this for anything between 10 and 30 minutes, or,

- Run up a flight of stairs. Now run or walk down. Keep doing this for anything between 10 and 30 minutes.

C. Advanced weight loss interval routine on hill or stair

This interval training is best done on a track.

- In the first lap, just walk the full circle on the track.

- Next, jog around the track – this is the second lap.

- Walk around the track once more – the third lap.

- Jog quickly (faster than the 1st lap) or run around the track – 4th lap.

Keep repeating this for 20 to 30 minutes.

For this, you do not even need a track…

- You can try doing this on a football field. Use just half the field, or,

- You can use the entire football field as a lap, or,

- You can use the neighborhood block as your lap.

This is for people in the advanced level, but are still close to intermediate…

- Walk the 1st lap at moderate speed.

- Jog the 2nd lap.

- Walk again at moderate speed for the 3rd lap.

- Sprint or run in the 4th lap.

Keep repeating this schedule for 10 to 30 seconds.

For those who are truly in the advanced stage, and ready for this…

- Walk or jog in the 1st lap.

- Jog or run in the 2nd lap.

- Walk or jog again in the 3rd lap.

- Jog or run faster or better still sprint in the 4th lap. Try to run so quickly as if a dog is chasing you.

Keep repeating this schedule for 10 to 30 minutes.

Beginner-To-Advanced Level 8-Week High Intensity Interval Program

Here is a HIIT program that can take you from a beginner to the advanced level in just 8 weeks.

- At the beginning, the work:rest ratio is 1:4. The total workout time in this phase is 15 minutes. This is your Phase 1.

- In Phase 2, the work time goes up, and this changes the ratio to 1:2. Total workout time in this phase is 17 minutes.

- The rest ratio goes down in Phase 3 by 50%. The ratio thus becomes 1:1. Total time of workout also goes up to 18.5 minutes.

- Phase 4 is the last stage. Here, the rest ratio goes down by 50% again. The ratio thus goes up to 2:1. The total workout time is now 20 minutes. When you have reached Phase 4, you will be in the advanced level of HIIT.

However, do keep in mind that this is just a suggested time. You may change it somewhat depending on how well your body is able to take the exercises. But remember to maintain the ratios. Go for it if you have to spend more than a couple of weeks in a particular stage, before moving up. Also, you can always jump up if any phase seems too easy to you.

The HIIT workouts can be done with tools like the jump rope. Or else, you may do sprinting, jumping jacks, or work on the stationary cycle.

Phase 1 (1:4): Weeks 1-2

- Do high intensity workout for 15 seconds.
- Low intensity workout or rest for 60 seconds.

Repeat this routine 10 times. Do a high intensity blast for 15 seconds after this.

Total exercise time – 14 minutes.

Phase 2 (1:2): Weeks 3-4

- Do high intensity workout for 30 seconds.
- Low intensity workout or rest for 60 seconds.

Repeat this routine 10 times. Do a high intensity blast for 30 seconds after this. Total exercise time – 17 minutes.

Phase 3 (1:1): Weeks 5-6

- Do high intensity workout for 30 seconds.
- Low intensity workout or rest for 30 seconds.

Repeat this routine 11 times. Do a high intensity blast for 30 seconds after this. Total exercise time – 18.5 minutes.

Phase 4 (2:1): Week 7-8

- Do high intensity workout for 30 seconds.
- Low intensity workout or rest for 15 seconds.

Repeat this routine 25 times. Do a high intensity blast for 30 seconds after this. Total exercise time – 20 minutes.

Chapter 6 : Treadmill Routines for Losing Belly Fat

Treadmills can help you improve your cardiovascular fitness and get rid of that stubborn belly fat as well. And they are among the safest and the most enjoyable exercises too. There are plenty of variations to keep you excited. Don't worry if you have not used a treadmill before. Nothing could be simpler.

Slow and Steady

Start it slowly. Your enthusiasm is worth praising, but if you are a beginner and if you speed off immediately, then you can get injured. It's a classic case of over-training. Try walking instead. Walk with a comfortable and slow pace for 5 to 10 minutes. Walk more briskly when you feel that your body can take a more intense workout. Continue for 30 minutes at this pace and then decrease your speed gradually. Remember – no sudden moves.

Add Some Incline

Add a little incline to your treadmill to make it a bit more intense. You will burn more calories and lose more fat at a higher intensity. Make sure that it's not so challenging that you are not able to do your 30 minutes on the machine. But warm up for 5-10 minutes before you do the incline. Don't keep your hands on the rails. Get support from the lower part of your body. Lower the incline after 30 minutes. Maintain a record of the degrees of incline, and increase it gradually.

Jogging

Try jogging after a couple of weeks. It can be a bit wobbly initially, but you'll get a hang of it soon enough. Once again, you should warm-up by walking for 5 to 10 minutes before jogging on your treadmill. Jogging will take up much more energy, and so start with 20 minutes. Increase this gradually.

Treadmill Rounds

A treadmill can make you lose a lot of weight. But it can get slightly boring after a while. This is where treadmill rounds can help you.

Here, you are essentially doing the treadmill to get your heart rate up, and then shifting your focus to floor exercises and weight training. Everything together works very well for you – you strengthen your muscles, boost your metabolism, and burn more fat. It stays interesting as well.

Do this for three rounds in a session. Something like this...

Round 1: The treadmill's speed should be at 10.5 miles/hour. Run for just 30 seconds, no more. Hop off the machine and do 10 pushups. Do 10 lunges after this. Repeat this twice.

Round 2: The treadmill's speed should be at 11 miles/hour. Run for just 30 seconds. Hop off and do 10 curls. Keep a weight in both your hands. Follow this up with 10 crunches. Repeat this twice.

Round 3: The treadmill's speed should be at 11.5 miles/hour. Run for 30 seconds. Do 10 squats and 10 pushups after this.

Those who are just starting off can do just a single repetition of each. Try to work your way up gradually.

Chapter 7 : Benefits of Weight Loss

There are plenty of benefits of weight loss. It's not just about looking better or being able to wear the old clothes that have become too tight. It has been medically proved that obesity can cause a number of health conditions. So by cutting your weight, you will be lowering your risks, and improving the quality of your life. Besides, a better-looking body can also give you the confidence to become more social, and perform better at the workplace as well.

Here are some benefits of weight loss.

1. You can prevent heart conditions and stroke – Heart disease and stroke are two of the most fatal conditions. They can cause death and disability. Those who are overweight have a higher chance of,

   - High Blood Pressure.

   - High cholesterol levels and blood fats (triglycerides). They can also cause heart diseases.

   - Angina – This is chest pain caused by reduced supply of oxygen to the heart. Obesity is a main cause of this.

   - Sudden death from stroke or heart disease without any symptom.

It has been seen that you can reduce your risk of developing stroke and heart disease by a great deal even with a 5% to 10% weight reduction. Triglycerides, cholesterol, blood pressure and heart function – everything improves.

2. Lose weight to prevent type 2 diabetes – Type 1 and type 2 diabetes can both cause long-term health complications that can bring down the quality of your life. It is assumed that obese people are two times more likely to have these issues as compared to others. Cut your weight, and you will be significantly reducing the chances of getting these conditions. But what if you already have type 1 or type 2 diabetes? You can improve your condition and even reduce medication with exercise and weight loss.

3. Reduce the risk of cancer – Researchers have discovered that many types of cancer are linked with obesity. For instance, obese women have a higher chance of cancer in the gallbladder, uterus, breast, colon, ovary and cervix. And men with a few extra pounds are at a higher risk of prostate, rectum and colon cancer. And of course, cancer can be fatal. Exercise, and change your diet to lose weight and reduce the risk.

4. Improves sleep apnea – Sleep apnea can make you snore heavily. This can even make you stop breathing for a short time. It can make you feel sleepy

during the day, and in extreme cases, may even lead to heart failure. You can reduce the risk significantly and even completely eliminate it by reducing weight.

5. <u>Reduce the risk of osteoarthritis</u> – Osteoarthritis is a joint disorder in the lower back, hips and knees. Those who are overweight have a higher risk, as the additional weight will increase the pressure on their joints. Weight loss can provide you relief from the associated pain.

6. <u>Gout</u> – High uric acid levels in the blood causes gout. This is also a joint disease. Those who are overweight are more likely to have this disease. Exercise and weight loss will give you relief. Some diets can trigger gout. So be careful about what you are eating.

7. <u>Gall bladder</u> – It has been seen that overweight people are more likely to have gallstones and gall bladder diseases. It can cause a lot of pain. Lose weight to reduce the risk.

Chapter 8: Forming Habits to Lose Weight

Most people are not able to lose weight easily, for one reason – it is very difficult to change old habits. So it's important to try and change the habits that made you overweight. Beat these habits, form new healthy ones, and you'll succeed.

How to Form Habits

You can form a habit by tying it to a trigger, and then by repeating it over and over again till the time it becomes automatic. But remember, you will have to make it long enough so that it can become automatic.

Here is a good habit plan...

1. Pick a new habit and replace the old one. Start with just a single habit, as this will be easier to follow. For instance, let us assume that you want to eat more green vegetables. So instead of all those sweets and chips, you can turn to carrots or cucumber for your snack. Again, if you check your email first thing in the morning, make it a point to go out for a walk for 30 minutes or doing some light exercises before doing so.

2. Keep your habit small. Often, many of us become too ambitious and do a lot to begin with. But that is rarely sustainable. We invariably we end up doing nothing. This is a trap. Pick up small habits instead that won't take up more than 5 minutes daily (such as running or walking). Give it type so that it becomes a part of your system. You can always extend it later.

3. Focus on enjoying the habit. You will surely quit if it feels too much like a sacrifice. The habit will become a reward if you are enjoying it.

4. Be accountable. Create a log of your new habit. Enter what you are doing everyday and share it with your friends and family. Let everybody know. This will make you more committed to your habit.

Stick to the above plan for long enough and it will become a part of your new lifestyle. That's how you can form new and healthier habits. Then pick up another habit and repeat the same process. You will soon be a changed person.

For instance, you can start with eating more vegetables. Start running or walking next. Go for water instead of soda. Go to the next step with body squats and pushups, and add some weights.

Chapter 9: Weight Loss Measuring Tools

Almost all of us, when we are trying to lose weight, keep looking at the scale every few days or weeks, but don't see much of a change. It can be so disheartening. There's a good reason for this – the scale does not tell the complete story.

Your body changes when you workout. Your heart works more efficiently. Your circulation gets better. These changes are all needed for weight loss, but you will rarely feel or see these changes. So how do you detect the changes?

Track the Body Fat

Body fat percentage gives you a more accurate picture than the scale. For instance, a bodybuilder might have 250 pounds, and yet just 8% body fat. The typical height-weight chart will mark the person "overweight".

By finding your body fat percentage, you can learn how much you need to shed, and can track your progress too. Here are some ways you can measure body fat percentage.

- Bioelectrical Impedance Scales

- Calipers

- Hydrostatic Weighing

- DEXA (dual energy X-ray absorptiometry)

Healthy women should have between 25% and 31% body fat, and for men it is between 18% and 25%.

- Check once a week or two weeks. Body fat will not go away overnight.

- Many gyms will one way of measuring body fat. But make the same person measure it every time. Different trainers can measure it in different ways. The results may not be comparable.

- If you are using the bioelectrical impedance scale, then make sure that you measure under the same circumstances every time. Skin temperature, food intake and hydration can all show different body fat measurements.

- Keep a log of the numbers.

Use the Scale

Yes, it's true that the scale won't give you the complete story always. Scales will measure everything – the weight of your bones, organs, muscle and fat. So you cannot tell whether you have actually lost fat or not.

However, that doesn't mean that the scale is completely useless. In fact, it is often the most convenient way to measure progress as the scale is available everywhere. Just make sure that you use the scale with the body fat percentage calculator. If you know both these numbers, you will be able to find out whether you are losing the right kind of weight – weight from your fat.

All you have to do is just multiply your weight by your body fat percentage. For instance, if you weigh 150 lbs, and have 21% body fat, then your total body fat is 31 lbs. so you know precisely where you stand.

Keep checking in this way to monitor your progress.

Conclusion

Thank you again for investing in yourself by downloading this book!

I hope you benefited from Weight Training for Weight Loss and were able to find out some very effective exercises for losing weight.

The next step is to start applying what you have learned and start doing these exercises. But let me warn you, be moderate in your approach to begin with. You can always scale up later. Add a few aerobics and interval training sessions to your weight training exercises, and you are sure to see that fat deposit going away in no time.

Thank you and I wish you the best of good luck!

If you received any value from this book, then I'd like to ask you for a favor. Would you be kind enough to leave a review for this book on amazon.com and/or like our Facebook page?

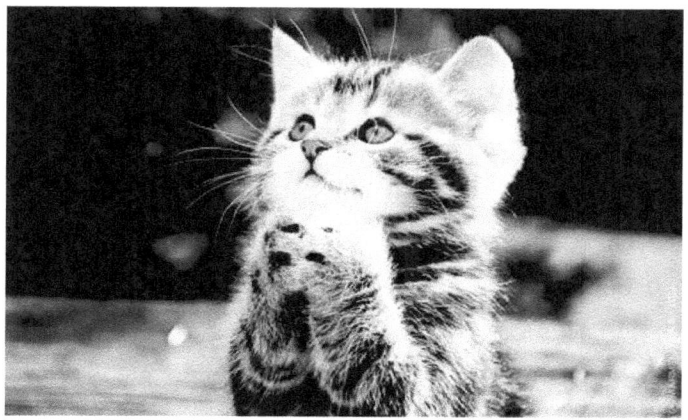

http://amzn.to/1eDPrOa

Leave a review at amazon.com now with one-click!

Like us on Facebook:

http://on.fb.me/1ORus09

Weight Training For Weight Loss:

How To Lose Weight And Build Muscle

John S. Edwards

Table Of Contents

Introduction

I want to thank you and congratulate you for downloading "Weight Training for Weight Loss: How to Lose Weight and Build Muscle"

This book contains proven steps and strategies on how to have a fit and well-toned body using weight training.

This is a quick, helpful and informative guide on weight training packed with tips, workout routine steps and handy advice on how to get the toned and fit body that you have been dreaming of using weight training!

We value your time, this book was created to pack in the most useful information targeting weight loss and muscle growth through weight training. All the content has been optimized to be simple and straight to the point. I truly hope you receive the most from it, and hope that you enjoy our work.

Chapter 1 – The Challenges of Getting Fit and Well-Toned

So you are planning to lose weight. Good for you! Today is the best day to start losing those extra pounds! With constant training and persistence, you will soon be able to successfully lose weight and do a lot of things that you were unable to do before! You will even get to wear clothes that were impossible to wear when you were still overweight! You can completely improve your physical, emotional and psychological well-being when you manage to lose weight. However, the journey to a new you is not going to be easy.

There is no miracle drug, wonder treatment or magic machine that could make you lose weight. You need to train and to train really hard. To be able to successfully get rid of unwanted fat and transform your body into a fit and well-toned vessel, you need to practice weight training.

You may have heard about weight training before or you may have heard so much about how successfully weight training has transformed shapeless, overweight and unsightly bodies into trim and lean ones. Weight training is a combination of strategies that will help you transform into a whole new you. If you are ready to live your dream, then let's start today. Let weight training get you that trim and fit body that you have been dreaming of in years!

Weight Training Defined

To be able to perform weight training, it is essential to learn what it is really about. We have described weight training as **NOT** a sure fire way to lose weight and to trim your body but rather it is composed of strategies aimed in losing and maintaining your weight, build stronger and leaner muscles and making you fit and healthy. Because it is a combination of these strategies, it could be very difficult to determine easily what the ideal weight training strategy is ideal for you.

Therefore, to paint a clearer picture of what weight training really is:

- **Weight training includes workout routines to build leaner and stronger muscles.**

  Workout routines that include the use of exercise equipment such as free weights and gym equipment. By correctly using these pieces of equipment, you will be able to slim down and tone different muscle groups. Routines should be done regularly with increasing resistance to take advantage of the benefits of different weight training equipment and to effectively trim and slim down in the least possible time.

- **Weight training involves the use of the right nutrients that you would get from food and supplements.**
  Even if you have managed to successfully tone down, it is important that you eat the right type of food to get nutrients that you need to develop stronger and leaner muscles. Combining weight training routines with the right diet could boost results. And determining the ideal diet plan is essential in achieving the best results of any weight training strategy.

- **Weight training is all about changing and adapting a new lifestyle to lose weight and keep weight off for good.**
  Another major component of weight loss and weight training is adapting an improved lifestyle. All your efforts to lose weight and to make your body trim and slim could be put to waste when you do not adapt a healthy lifestyle. This is no easy matter since you are used to doing things in a particular way; changing could definitely be very hard to do. For instance, you may be used to eating out during lunch or you tend to drink alcohol especially beer after work.
  Eating healthy food that you have prepared at home could be a drastic change and you may need to spend time preparing your healthy food too. Saying no to a drink after work is a very difficult thing to do. Having self-control allows you to take matters into your hands and change your lifestyle into something better and something healthier.

- **Weight training is a planned approach to weight loss and in every training regimen, careful planning is done** (this will be discussed in detail in the later chapters).
  Planning makes every endeavor successful and this is why detailed planning will make your weight loss strategies easier to achieve and helps you focus on your goals better. Planning takes careful consideration of your present situation and this includes how

much you currently weigh, your state of health, your level of activity and the tools or materials that you have access to. Plans should be systematic and flexible to allow you to adjust your responses to different situations easily.

Every person is different and therefore no weight training strategy is the same. Each person has his own goals too and creating a goal that will work for your needs is very important.

Chapter 2 – Components of Weight Training Using Training Equipment

When you look up weight training strategies online, the most popular definition would be about a combination of workout routines that use a set of weights. Equipment such as free weights is very important to define your body and these are dumbbells, barbells and kettlebells. There are also routines that include the use of weight training machines such as those found in gyms. When it comes to using equipment and devices, the following components of weight training are very important:

1. **Increasing Load Resistance** – an important part of weight training using free weights and training machines is increasing the resistance that your body or specifically your muscles are used to. If you are used to lifting a 10-pound dumbbell, then you should apply more resistance about three to five pounds of weight. This strategy will not just avoid plateaus but will also improve your muscle strength. A good rule of thumb is that you should lift enough weight that you will be able to lift to complete a desired number of repetitions. You should be able to complete your last repetition with difficulty but still in good form.

   This is not just applicable using free weights but will also apply to using gym equipment that is used for weight training such as bench presses. Slowly increasing your resistance will allow you to improve your muscle strength as well as your form in the long run. It could also apply to cycling, walking, running and all other activities.

2. **Workout Progression** - your weight training workouts should increase in intensity as regularly as possible. This is very important so that you could avoid plateaus. The results of your workouts should be recorded and the selection of next workout regimen and level of resistance should be according to the results of the final repetition. Just like increasing load resistance, progression also

applies to other types of exercises and this time, load progression can be done by increasing the amount of weight that you can muster, changing the number of repetitions that you usually do, changing sets and exercises

Changes such as increasing load resistance may be done on a weekly or monthly basis.

3. **Specific in Training** – weight training involves a variety of strategies; which sometimes are very confusing for someone that has never tried it before. Experts believe that the best way for weight training to be effective is to first focus on one part of your training and then the rest or as you go along. For instance, if one of your goals is to increase muscle strength then you should train for this using a program that has been designed to fulfill your goals. To boost muscle strength, a combination of circuit training and training using heavier weights are recommended to totally improve muscle strength.

4. **Have Adequate Rest and Recovery Periods** – continuous training could significantly increase your muscle mass, strength and tone however may place you at risk for injuries and muscle wear and tear. Therefore, every weight training strategy, no matter how simple or how complicated this may be should have adequate rest periods. It is during rest time that the body is able to regain its strength and it is able to repair injured cells and tissues. Our body is a smart machine it knows when it is tired and when it needs to have a break. Having ample rest periods is essential to any kinds of training.

Weight training is all about using a variety of weight training strategies and at the same time being aware of your diet, lifestyle and your rest periods. When all these are carefully considered, you will be able to lose weight, trim down and become leaner and stronger in no time at all.

Chapter 3 – Types of Weight Training

Bodybuilding Weight Training

In bodybuilding weight training there is only one goal and that is to make muscle groups bigger. Bodybuilders train for different reasons; this could be for competition, to simply improve their form or to buff their bodies for an event. The most common strategies that bodybuilders adapt is lifting weights in the 8 to 12 repetitions range and mostly, only one type of muscle group is trained per day in a week.

- Muscles look larger, defined and bulky

- Although muscles look larger and more defined, these are not stronger

Powerlifting Weight Training

As opposed to bodybuilding weight training, powerlifting training is preparing the muscles to make them stronger. The appearance of the muscles is not important in a powerlifter but instead the strength and the ability of the muscles to sustain stress are more important than aesthetics.

- Muscles look lean and trim

- Muscles are amazingly strong and usually tested in powerlifting events

- The appearance and strength of muscles could only last for a few repetitions especially in lifting very heavy weights

Circuit Weight Training

Circuit training is a different type of weight training wherein you create a number of exercises in quick successions. This involves lifting light weights in multiple repetitions. Exercises are done without any kind of rest in between therefore a person could perform 20 bench presses, shoulder presses and squats without resting. The aim of circuit weight training is to burn fat and at the same time defines and strengthens muscles.

This type of weight training is usually done by athletes and fighters since during actual performance or as they perform their particular sport, there is little to no rest in between rounds. For instance, in a mixed martial arts fight, the athlete needs to endure a lot of stress and pressure as he fights another fighter in the octagon. He may have little rest in between rounds. Circuit training makes the body ready for this kind of stress.

- Muscles look large, trim and defined.

- Muscles are strong and can endure continuous stress.

- The appearance and the strength of muscles last for a longer period of time and therefore you could last and endure stress longer.

Isometric Weight Training

In isometric weight training, you will be training your muscles to endure physical strain and stamina. The most common strategy is holding a weight, a dumbbell or a barbell, in a particular position for a given number of time without moving your arm or leg. The purpose of isometric training is to improve your stamina in certain situations where you need to hold your position. Rock climbers need to hold positions to be able to climb higher. He steps from one crevice to another and holds onto something or places his foot on a foothold and maintains a position so that he could move up.

- Muscles look large, firm and trim

- Muscles are strong and can endure longer amounts of stress and strain

- Muscles can maintain different positions for a long period of time

High- Volume Weight Training

This kind of weight training is very similar to bodybuilding training since you only develop one muscle group at a time. Muscles in bodybuilding training look strong, lean and defined but are not necessarily strong. In high-volume training, the muscles are also trained to endure stress to make them look larger and at the same time resilient to stress for a longer period of time.

High-volume weight training programs usually involves performing a type of exercise and one kind of weight for multiple sets and times. For example, you will lift a 15 - pound weight this week for 10 times and for 10 sets and then increase the amount of weight week after week. In the process your muscles become stronger and more defined.

- Muscles are large, firm and trim

- Muscles are strong and can endure stress for a longer period of time

As you can see, there are different kinds of weight training strategies. Each one has its advantages and disadvantages and possible uses; choosing the ideal training plan is essential in achieving exactly what you want.

Chapter 4 – The Benefits of Weight Training

Weight training has a lot of benefits not just physical but also psychological and emotional benefits too. Through weight training, you will be able to reap the following benefits:

1. **You will have an attractive body**

    There is no doubt that you will have a wonderful body by the time you are finished with weight training. You will be able to become leaner and fit when you regularly indulge with weight training.

2. **You will be able to lose weight**

    You will be able to reduce your weight with circuit training. You will burn calories and thus help you get rid of unwanted fat to finally become healthier and trim. Being obese and overweight will make you more susceptible to different illnesses. Medical conditions such as hypertension, cardiac problems, and increased cholesterol levels could be due to being obese. Indulging in weight training will help you get rid of unwanted fat and reduce the likelihood of suffering from these conditions in the future.

3. **You will be able to strengthen your muscles and improve your endurance and stamina**

    Powerlifting, bodybuilding, isometric and high-intensity weight training all help to improve your muscle strength. Although results are in varying degrees, you will have better and more powerful muscle abilities in such a way that you will be able to lift heavier weights over a longer period of time and even manage to maintain a stressful position in an extended period of time.

4. **You will be able to improve your self-esteem**

There is no doubt that you will have improved self-esteem when you see the amazing results of weight training! So let's start now!

Chapter 5 – Creating a Weight Training Plan

As mentioned earlier, a weight training plan is important to be able to determine exactly what your goals are. It does not matter if you are new to weight training or you have done this kind of training before. It takes a careful assessment of what your current needs are as well as your current situation to be able to formulate a suitable plan. Sit down and open your mind; this is a very important part of weight training and should be taken very seriously.

1. Determine your actual goal. Possible goals are to lose weight, to increase muscle size, to increase muscle strength, to improve muscle endurance, to improve stamina or to improve strength to be able to perform sports or physical activities. Your goal determines the type of weight training strategy that you should use.

2. After you have a clear picture of your goal, take time to create a feasible statement for it. This statement is something that will describe your goal and something that will make it achievable. Simply saying that you want to increase your muscle strength could be very vague. A better goal statement would be being able to lift a particular amount of weight after a certain amount of time or days. You could say that "lifting a 50-pound barbell after four weeks to get ready for a powerlifting competition" is feasible enough.

3. Assess your current physical situation. Do you have certain issues that you need to resolve?

- Find out your current weight and height and use these numbers to find out if you are overweight or not. There are several ways to determine if you have a normal weight, if you are overweight or if you are obese and using your weight and your height is one of the most basic techniques.

A good way to measure your weight is to use a reliable and accurate weighing scale. Wear only your undergarments and remove any footwear. Measure your weight in the morning before you eat breakfast. Take your measurements on the same time of the day, every day and be sure to remember these tips.

- Calculate your **BMR or basal metabolic rate**. Your BMR will determine the amount of calories that you burn while at rest. This amount of calories is needed by your body to perform basic functions and this does not include the number of calories that you will use for exercise and physical activities. When you have an idea of your BMR, you will know how many calories you will need to burn to be able to lose weight.

If you plan to use weight training to lose weight, then you should first determine your BMR. The formula goes this way:

- For women **(4.35 x body weight in pounds) + (4.7 x height in inches) - (4.68 x age) + 655.**

- For men, the formula is **(6.25 x body weight in pounds) + (12.7 x height in inches) - (6.76 x age) + 66.**

The result is the number of calories you should burn per day were so you to remain sedentary and do nothing more than sit or lie down.

- Take your measurements. This is very important if you plan to improve your muscle size as well as your strength then you should take measurements of the muscle groups that you want to improve. For instance, measuring your biceps is a must if you want to improve this muscle group, taking measurements of your chest will help you create a goal to make this part of your body larger and firmer while measuring your midsection will help you create a starting point on your goals to reduce and firm this troublesome area.

A good way to measure the body part that you wish to measure is to use a reliable measuring tape. Just like taking your weight, measure on the same time of day. You may also take photos of your figure to emphasize what you want to achieve. Take a selfie pose while facing the mirror and make sure you flaunt the body part that you wish to improve!

- Consider any physical conditions that you may have. These could directly or indirectly affect the way you train. For instance, you have high blood pressure or diabetes; these conditions could definitely limit the way you work out. Considering the help of your doctor in determining the right exercise regimen will assist you in creating the most suitable training goals.

4. Consider the amount of time that you are willing to spare in working out is also important. If you are a very busy person, then you could rely on a weight training regimen that will give you faster results in just a few minutes of training each day. If you have a lot of time to spare, then you could indulge in long term exercise training to be able to come up with lasting results.

5. Consider your location or the place where you plan to train. Here are some important points:

    - It is recommended that you train in a facility where there is complete weight training equipment.

    - The gym should have an in-house expert and professional trainer should you need help.

    - The gym should be accessible from where you live. You should select a local gym so you will be able to commit to daily workouts rain or shine.

- The gym should have training programs to help you with your goals. These could be circuit training programs, bodybuilding programs and so on.

But if you want to train at home then this is possible as well! However, you should have patience, have a clear image of your goals and be able to train every day.

6. Finally, your goal should include a feasible date or time when you plan to achieve it. Experts also suggest creating short term goals.

When you have finished all these, it's time to put your plan to the test! You will now be able to start your weight training regimen as soon as you are ready!

Chapter 6 – Weight Training Workouts

Basic Weight raining Workouts (BONUS)

It is time to learn about basic weight training workouts. These are basic workout strategies that you will possibly use for different types of weight training. You may combine these to create the ideal training regimen to achieve your goals however the following is a sample of weight training that is developed for beginners. This is a full body routine that uses a systematic regimen of different workouts that will improve your upper body, lower body, your midsection and your back.

The Full Body Routine (BONUS)

This is a workout routine that will cover for three days and is used by beginners so they could become more familiar with the exercises since they will be repeating these a number of times in a week. Beginners actually experience more gains when they train less and therefore these routines are the best one to start with. Each routine should be followed with a period of rest. This period may vary and a beginner usually takes around 30 minutes to an hour to rest and adjust before he could do another type of routine. As you go along, you will find that you may hardly think of resting and even would like to proceed to the next routine at once. This is okay but you still need to remember to rest adequately especially when you are new to the routines,

DAY 1:

- Start with *squats* around 4 sets of 8 repetitions. Also known as Olympic squats or barbell full squats; you will perform squats with the use of a barbell. This exercise targets the quadriceps, calves, glutes and hamstrings.

  1. Stand with your feet apart and your hands to each sides. The barbell is in front of you.

2. Take the barbell and lift it over your head and carefully pass it over your head and hold it over your shoulders. Your legs to form a squat to allow you to carry the barbell over your head.

3. Do 8 repetitions each time keeping your chin up and your hips and knees together.

4. Finish the routine by passing the barbell over your head and placing it back on the ground.

5. Perform 4 sets and 8 repetitions, afterwards take a rest.

- *Barbell bench presses* around 4 sets of 8 repetitions. Bench presses target the chest, shoulders and triceps.

  1. Use a standard bench to perform your presses. Ready the barbell on the rack. Lie down with your back against the bench and keep your foot on the floor.

  2. Now start gripping the barbell. Your palms should be facing outward and gripping the barbell on each end near the plate.

  3. Start making a press. Slowly lift the barbell from the rack to as far up as it can go and then with one or two counts place the barbell back on the rack. After about a second, proceed with lifting the weight again and then placing it back on the rack. Repeat this in 4 sets of 8 repetitions.

- *Pull – ups* around 4 sets of 8 repetitions using dumbbells with gradually-increasing weights. This routine targets the lats, biceps and the middle back.

  1. Stand or sit with your legs apart and with one or two dumbbells on each hand.

  2. With your back straight and your feet apart, slowly bring one dumbbell from the floor to your chin and then place it back on the floor.

3. Repeat for 8 repetitions of 4 sets.

- *Barbell curls* around 4 sets of 8 repetitions using a barbell with gradually-increasing weights. This targets the biceps and forearms.

    1. Stand with your feet apart and your back straight. Place the barbell in front on the floor.

    2. Bend with your knees to hold the barbell and to raise it towards your chest. Your hand should have the palms facing you to fully lift the weight without difficulty.

    3. Lift the barbell so that it touches your chest area and then place it back on the floor. Remember to bend your legs to lift and to place the weights back on the floor.

    4. Repeat this for 8 repetitions and 4 sets.

- *Standing military press* around 4 sets of 8 repetitions. This is extending the barbell over your head. Barbells are used with gradually –increasing weights. This targets the shoulders and triceps.

    1. Stand with your feet apart and your back straight. Lift the barbell before you with your palms facing you.

    2. Lift the barbell over your head and then place this over your head. Go back to the original position to bring the barbell down.

DAY 2: Rest Day

Rest days are important since your body needs to recover from any strain and stress. This is also a great time for your muscles to get acquainted with the stress that it has received. The body also naturally repairs tissues and this is also done when you are not working out.

DAY 3:

- *Deadlifts* around 5 sets of 5 repetitions. Barbell deadlifts fortifies the lower back, calves, forearms, glutes, middle back and the quadriceps.

  1. Start by standing while your feet are apart and your back is straight. The barbell is in front of you.

  2. Bend with your knees to lift the barbell with your hands on both ends of the equipment. Your palms should be facing you to fully lift the barbell efficiently.

  3. Lift up to your waistline and then place it back down with bended knees.

  4. Repeat this for 5 repetitions and for 5 sets.

- *Bent over rows* around 5 sets of 5 repetitions using a heavy barbell. This strengthens the middle back, biceps, lats and shoulders.

  1. Similar to a deadlift you will need to stand with your feet apart and your back straight.

  2. Lift the barbell from the ground to your waist level. But instead of just bending your knees to raise the barbell, bend forward to provide more lifting force. Remember that you are lifting a heavier barbell compared to other routines and therefore you need more help in lifting this up.

  3. Place the heavy barbell back onto the floor. Repeat these steps for 5 repetitions and 5 sets.

- *Lateral raises* around 5 sets of 5 repetitions using a dumbbell. This routine strengthens the shoulder muscles.

  1. Stand with your feet apart and your back straight. Dumbbells must be on each hand.

  2. Raise your upper arms and then lift the dumbbell laterally from your body. You may perform this using the right arm first and then the left. Your palms should be facing the side of your body as you lift the weights laterally.

  3. Perform 5 repetitions and 5 sets. Move slowly but surely to avoid any injuries.

- *Dumbbell triceps extensions* 5 sets of 5 repetitions use a dumbbell. This routine improves the triceps muscles.

  1. Use a moderately heavy dumbbell. Start the routine with the dumbbell at the back of your head. Hold it with both hands on the handle.

  2. Lift the dumbbell till it is positioned on top of your head and then return to the initial position.

  3. Repeat these steps for 5 times for 5 sets. End the routine by carefully placing the barbell back on the floor by passing it from the back of your head to the front and then finally to the floor.

- *Hammer curls* 5 sets of 5 repetitions using dumbbells. This routine improves your biceps.

  1. Stand up with your feet apart and your back straight. Place a dumbbell on each hand

2. Lift the dumbbell towards your chest area alternately. Your palms should be facing you as you grip the dumbbells efficiently.

3. Repeat this for 5 times and 5 sets. Place the dumbbells back on the floor carefully by bending your knees and your back.

Day 4:

- *Lunges* around 3 sets of 12 repetitions. These improves the quadriceps, calves, glutes and hamstrings

  1. Stand straight with a dumbbell on both hands.

  2. Step forward using your right leg and your foot left behind with your body lowered. Maintain your balance and keep your torso upright.

  3. Use the heel of your foot to push up and to return to the starting position.

  4. Do the recommended movements for the arms such as placing the dumbbell on your chest.

  5. Repeat the steps using the other leg. Repeat for 12 times and in 3 sets.

- *Dips or triceps dips* around 3 sets and 12 repetitions. This strengthens the triceps, shoulders and chest muscles. You will use an exercise machine for this routine.

  1. Start by facing the exercise machine and hold each of the bars with your hands.

  2. Use these bars to lift your body off the floor. The equipment usually has bars that jut out along the midsection and therefore you will hang using these bars

for a particular amount of time and repetitions. Holding your body will help improve muscle resistance to stress and strain.

3. Another variation is to lift until both your arms are extended. This lifts your body off the floor for a great deal of height and then lowering to the original position.

4. Repeat for 12 times and for 3 sets. Carefully lower your body to the original position and step off the machine.

- *Chin ups* around 3 sets of 12 repetitions. This improves the lats, biceps and forearms. You will use an exercise machine to perform this routine.

  1. Stand in front of an exercise equipment and grab the handle to raise the weights with each hand.

  2. Inhale and pull the handles till these are close to your chin.

  3. Exhale and release the handle to lower the weights carefully.

  4. Repeat this routine for 12 times and for 3 sets.

- *Push press* around 3 sets of 12 repetitions using kettlebells. This improves the calves, quadriceps, triceps and calves.

  1. Place a kettlebell on each hand and stand straight with your feet apart.

  2. Lift the kettlebell until it is on your shoulder and then rotate your wrist to allow the weights to be placed on your shoulders.

  3. Perform squats for 12 repetitions and 3 sets. Afterwards, carefully lower the kettlebells to the ground.

- *Seated calf raises* around 3 sets of 12 repetitions using a weight training machine. This routine improves the calves.

  1. Sit on the weight training machine and place your feet on the foot rest.

  2. Extend your legs to lift the weight and then slowly lower this to its original position by returning to an original seated position.

  3. Repeat for 12 times and for 3 sets. You may use this routine for isometric training by lifting the weight and then holding the position for a few minutes.

- *Plate twists* uses only the barbell or dumbbell plates around 3 sets of 12 repetitions. This routine firms the abdominals.

  1. Hold the barbell or dumbbell plates with both hands. Sit on the floor with both your feet extended in front.

  2. With your hands on the plate, twist your body. When the plate is on your right, your legs and knees should be on the opposite side.

  3. Repeat this for 12 times and for 3 sets.

As you can see, all these routines may be enhanced using very simple techniques.

- You can increase the amount of weight that you are holding by simply adding more plates to your barbell or using a suitable dumbbell weight.

- You can increase the number of repetitions as well as the number of sets that you do to increase resistance.

- Instead of just bending over and lifting the barbell over your head, try to hold the barbell for a few seconds to improve muscle resistance to stress.

- You may also perform the workout routines every day instead of having a rest day however this is not recommended since the body needs to recuperate and repair itself.

- You can adjust settings on weight training machines to increase the height of the seat or the equipment.

- You can train continuously without any rest in between techniques. The more you strain your body the more it will learn to adapt to this stress. You will find yourself stronger, fitter, leaner and more defined in no time at all.

Simple Weight Training Tips

Now that you have learned the simplest and the most basic weight training strategies it is time to find out a few more simple tips on how to be closer to your goal. No matter what goal you have (weight loss, increased muscle size or increased muscle strength) you need the following tips.

- **You are what you eat**

  o Now that you are building muscles and making them stronger, you need to consume the right kind of food. The best foods to eat during these periods are foods rich in high quality protein. Not only will protein help you lose weight since it is harder to digest proteins but it will also help you bulk up. Fantastic foods that will help you become leaner and healthier are fish, lean meats, eggs, and seafood, milk, poultry and milk products. You may also take supplements such as protein shakes and protein bars. It is best to consult a specialist to help you select the best supplements for weight loss and muscle gain.

- **Lifestyle changes**

- If you smoke, then this is the best time to quit. Smoking affects the way your blood delivers nutrients and oxygen to your body tissues including your muscles and therefore quitting will help you bulk up a lot.

- Reduce alcohol intake to help improve your health. Alcohol also affects the body's ability to remove waste products and removing wastes and toxins are important in maintaining the ideal weight and health.

- Avoid eating out instead cook and prepare your own healthy foods.

- Be more active. Move about, enroll in any weight training course, dance, take up sports or run. There are so many different ways to become more active and these will help you significantly in improving your figure, form and your health.

- **Stress management**

  - Learn how to manage stress to help you think positively when you train. There will never be anything good out of being stressed and anxious, you will only be less effective in making decisions. There are many ways to manage stress, you can exercise, take up sports, do yoga, meditate, read, listen to music or talk to friends. The more you are able to handle your stress better the more you will be able to train without interruptions and will also help you visualize your goals.

- **Rest and recovery**

  Never overlook rest and recovery periods. As mentioned, it is during this time when the body is able to rest and recover from stress, injuries and any kind of pain. Resting at least a day is important in people who are new to weight training and although you may find it easy after a few weeks, you will still need to rest to cope with future workout routines which will be more strenuous than ever.

Conclusion

Thank you again for downloading "Weight Training for Weight Loss: How to Lose Weight and Build Muscle"

The next step is to actively follow the information here and you are sure to see result quickly, I guarantee it. We truly want to see you succeed in achieving a trimmer and slimmer you!

I hope we are able to help you reach your fitness goals. If you have any questions or would like to contact us, please do so in our Facebook Fan Page, we would love to help you in your journey towards a greater body.

http://on.fb.me/1UJYqom

Thank you and stay motivated.

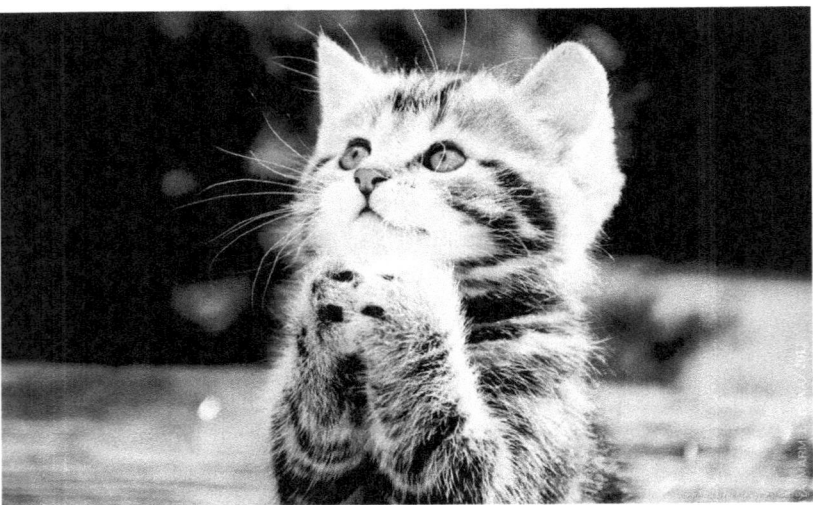

If you gain or learned anything from "Weight Training for Weight Loss", It would be amazing to receive an Amazon Review from you.

Amazon Review Link:

http://amzn.to/1mrY5DX

Thank You!

I want to start off by saying thank you for choosing to read one of my books. I know there are millions of other books out there and how valuable your time is so I am extremely grateful that you took the time out of your day to read my book.

I also want to quickly explain to you that you are getting 2 books within this 1 book you purchased! I wanted to give you this extra book as my way of saying thank you to you!

All you need to do is go back to the table of contents and you will see the 2nd book you are getting along with this one!

If you would like to go to the table of contents and check out the 2nd book

>>CLICK HERE<<

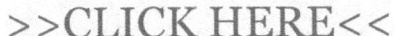

If you would like to go back to the beginning of the book

>>CLICK HERE<<